# Chair Yoga for Seniors

## Gentle Poses for Rejuvenation

Judith Delgado

# CONTENTS


Introduction ...................................................................................1

What Is Chair Yoga? .........................................................................3

Benefits ..........................................................................................4

Why Chair Yoga? ..............................................................................5

What are the Benefits of Chair Yoga? ...................................................8

   Examples of Chair Yoga Poses ......................................................10

Precautions ...................................................................................11

Particular Concerns Regarding Health ................................................12

Equipment ....................................................................................13

   Clothing ...................................................................................13

   Yoga mat ..................................................................................13

Safety ..........................................................................................14

General Tips ..................................................................................14

Get Yourself Warmed Up. .................................................................16

Warming different parts ...................................................................17

   1. Feet .....................................................................................17

   2. Calves ..................................................................................18

   3. Knees ...................................................................................18

   4. Thighs ..................................................................................18

   5. Belly ....................................................................................19

   6. Arms ....................................................................................19

   7: The Head and the Neck .............................................................19

   8. Tapping on the chest ................................................................20

   9. Rubbing the Heart ...................................................................20

Getting Started ..............................................................................21

Grounding....................................................................21

Meditation .................................................................22

Exercises for the Breath.............................................23

Breathing through each nostril in turn ....................23

Three Core Components of Chair Yoga......................26

Community.................................................................27

Compassion ...............................................................28

Circulation ................................................................29

½ Sun Salutations from a Seated Position ...............30

Flexion and Extension (Better Known as Cat/Cow)....31

Turn both to the right and left...................................31

Lateral bend The Right and the Left.........................32

Shoulder Movements to the Front and Back.............32

Wrists........................................................................33

Hips/Ankles ..............................................................33

Warrior 2 Seated .......................................................35

Uttkatasana...............................................................36

The "Down Dog".........................................................37

Plank.........................................................................37

Figure 4.....................................................................38

Savasana ...................................................................39

Warming up ...............................................................40

Mountain Pose ..........................................................41

The breath..................................................................41

Shoulder Shrugs........................................................42

Raise your arms above using both of them. .............44

Knee Swings ..............................................................44

Exercises for the Ankles Using Both Legs ................45

Neck Bend..................................................................46

Neck Turns ................................................................................47

Beginner Program .....................................................................48

Mountain Pose ...........................................................................48

The breath...................................................................................49

Side Neck Bend...........................................................................50

Neck Turns ...................................................................................50

Shoulder Shrugs ..........................................................................51

Wrist Circles.................................................................................51

Raise your arms above using both of them................................52

Knee Swings .................................................................................53

Complete a set of ankle circles with both legs .........................54

Shoulder Twists and Rolls...........................................................54

Bending Forward While Maintaining a Straight Back .............55

Alternating Arm Raises ...............................................................56

Twist of the Torso with Arms Raise...........................................57

Turning of the torso when the arms are extended out to the sides
.......................................................................................................58

Lean to the side of your body while raising both arms. ..........59

Single Arm and Leg Raises..........................................................59

Single-Leg Raises ........................................................................60

Single Knee Raises ......................................................................60

Point and Flex with a Single-Leg................................................61

Single-Leg Ankle Circles.............................................................62

Each of the Legs Points and Bends ...........................................62

Heel Raises...................................................................................63

Toe Raises ....................................................................................63

Toe Squeeze .................................................................................64

Everything on the Table .............................................................65

Deep Relaxation Pose .................................................................65

Increasing the time .................................................................67

The breath..............................................................................68

Side Neck Bend........................................................................68

Neck Turns...............................................................................69

Shoulder Shrugs ......................................................................70

Rings on the Wrists..................................................................70

Raise your arms above using both of them .............................71

Knee Swings.............................................................................71

Complete a set of ankle circles with both legs .......................72

Rolls with the Hands on the Shoulders ...................................73

Shoulder Twists and Rolls........................................................73

Bending Forward While Maintaining a Straight Back ..............74

Alternating Arm Raises ............................................................75

Extend(ing) Their Arms Palm Rotation ...................................75

Extend(ing) Their Arms Hand Squeeze ...................................76

Twist of the Torso with Arms Raise..........................................77

Turning of the torso when the arms are extended out to the sides
.................................................................................................78

Back Bend.................................................................................79

Lean to the side of your body while raising both arms .............79

Twist in the Chair.....................................................................80

Single Arm and Leg Raises.......................................................81

Single Knee Raises ...................................................................82

Point and Flex with a Single-Leg..............................................83

Single-Leg Ankle Circles...........................................................83

Each of the Legs Points and Bends ..........................................84

Heel Raises...............................................................................85

Toe Raises ................................................................................85

Toe Squeeze .............................................................................86

Everything on the Table ........................................................86

Position for Deep Relaxation ...............................................87

Intermediate Level of Practice ...................................................89

The breath.........................................................................91

Side Neck Bend.................................................................91

Neck Turns........................................................................92

Shoulder Shrugs ...............................................................93

Rings on the Wrists...........................................................93

Raise your arms above using both of them......................94

Knee Swings......................................................................94

Complete a set of ankle circles with both legs ................95

Rolls with the Hands on the Shoulders............................96

Shoulder Twists and Rolls.................................................96

Bending Forward While Maintaining a Straight Back ................97

Arm Raises interspersed with Weighted Exercises ................98

Rotation of the trunk while holding weights in extended arms ..99

Exercise for the Side of the Body Using Weights ................100

Bicep Curls with Weights, Performing Alternating Arms..........101

Raise your arms and legs individually using weights. ...............101

With weights, do single knee raises? ...............................102

Sit-stand up......................................................................103

Point and Flex with a Single-Leg.....................................104

Single-Leg Ankle Circles..................................................104

Each of the Legs Points and Bends .................................105

Back Bend.........................................................................106

Twist in the Chair.............................................................106

Extend(ing) Their Arms Perform palm rotations while holding weights.......................................................................107

Single-Leg Lifts with Weights..........................................108

Heel Raises.................................................................109

Toe Raises ..............................................................109

Toe Squeeze ...........................................................110

Everything Dependent upon the Weights................110

Position for Deep Relaxation..................................111

Increasing the time ....................................................113

The breath...........................................................113

Side Neck Bend......................................................114

Neck Turns ............................................................115

Shoulder Shrugs ....................................................115

Raise your arms above using both of them.............117

Knee Swings...........................................................117

Complete a set of ankle circles with both legs .......118

Rolls with the Hands on the Shoulders..................119

Shoulder Twists and Rolls......................................119

Bending Forward While Maintaining a Straight Back .............120

Arm Raises interspersed with Weighted Exercises .....................121

Rotation of the trunk while holding weights in extended arms 122

Exercise for the Side of the Body Using Weights .........................123

Bicep Curls with Weights, Performing Alternating Arms..........124

Raise your arms and legs individually using weights................124

With weights, do single knee raises? .....................125

Sit-stand up............................................................126

Point and Flex with a Single-Leg...........................127

Each of the Legs Points and Bends ........................128

Back Bend...............................................................129

Twist in the Chair ..................................................130

Extend(ing) Their Arms Perform palm rotations while holding
weights...................................................................130

Single-Leg Lifts with Weights..................................131

Heel Raises........................................................132

Toe Raises ........................................................132

Toe Squeeze ......................................................133

Everything Dependent upon the Weights..............133

Position for Deep Relaxation .............................134

Positions While Standing....................................136

1. Forward Fold ................................................136

2. Raised Knee Balance.....................................137

3. Hip Half-Circle .............................................138

4. On Your Tiptoes............................................139

7. From the Ground Up to Standing....................143

8. Tree .............................................................144

9. Warrior I .....................................................146

You can do this anywhere! .................................148

Gather your friends ..........................................151

feeling a lot better?..........................................154

Healthy diet.....................................................156

Meditation .......................................................158

Volunteering.....................................................160

Connection to both the community and society ...163

Calming Down ..................................................166

The Palming .....................................................166

Rest and Repose at the End...............................167

*"And in the end, it's not the years in your life that count. It's the life in your years."* —Abraham Lincoln, U.S. President.

# Introduction

Getting older is a blessing since it brings experience, knowledge, and poise. On the other hand, worry and tension, in addition to other chronic illnesses, might arise during this transitional aging period. Yoga may now be practiced even by those with physical restrictions, thanks to chair yoga. It makes it possible for seniors to stretch every part of their body while sitting down, which is particularly beneficial for those who have restricted movement and are in danger of falling. It is very uncommon for older citizens to have discomfort in one region. As a result, they cease engaging in physical activity altogether for other areas of their bodies. People who wish to keep active and preserve their physical and mental health will find that chair yoga is an excellent option. These low-impact activities ease the discomfort and stiffness in the joints and muscles.

The essential benefit is that older people may learn to control their breathing, lowering their tension and anxiety levels.

Through the use of gravity and one's body weight as resistance, Hatha yoga encourages balance across the whole body. The sequences include extended posture holding, allowing you to concentrate on how your body is aligned. During the session, you will have the opportunity to loosen up your muscles, minimize any feelings of stiffness, and stretch out. This works at striking a balance between the negative aspects of the physical body, namely the front and rear, left and right, and top and bottom. The use of a chair provides support for leg strengthening postures as well as balancing exercises. Practicing yoga regularly helps you develop the physical and mental fortitude you need to tackle the more challenging elements of everyday life.

Contrary to what you may see on Instagram, practicing yoga does not include contorting your body into the shape of a pretzel or standing on your head. It is about establishing a connection between the mind and the breath. The good news is that this applies to everyone, even elderly citizens interested in reaping the advantages of chair yoga for seniors.

As a yoga teacher who works with seniors who live in assisted-living facilities, I've seen how adding chairs to the practice can help a senior's mood, mobility, and a whole host of other aspects of their lives. All of a sudden, it feels like almost anybody could do yoga. To put it another way, it is the essence of yoga.

# What Is Chair Yoga?

The mild practice of yoga known as "chair yoga" is performed either while seated in a chair or standing with the assistance of a chair. Chair yoga doesn't need any specialist equipment or a significant amount of room, so almost everyone can do it, and it's also quite flexible in terms of where it may be done. For example, classes or routines on chair yoga could include light stretching, self-massage, meditation, breathing exercises, or any mix of these components.

Is chair yoga beneficial for older people? Yes! Chair yoga is an ancient form of yoga that involves doing traditional poses while seated on a chair. Although sitting on a chair for exercise is most often associated with elderly populations, it benefits individuals of all ages and levels of ability.

Doing yoga while seated on a chair makes the practice more approachable, provides additional support, and lowers the chance of falling while exercising. Additionally, it may aid with alignment, making it easier to do poses usually done on the floor while sitting in a chair.

However, it would help if you did not get the wrong

idea. There are many different styles of chair yoga to choose from. In addition, there is a wide range of degrees of difficulty; thus, you must choose a course guided by an experienced teacher that is both low-key and risk-free.

# Benefits

In my experience, chair yoga is the sort of yoga that is most beneficial for seniors. This is primarily because it helps create confidence and is more approachable to many individuals. Therefore, whether you are above the age of 60 or physically constricted, like some of my students, there are chair yoga postures that will likely benefit you.

In addition, the yoga positions described below are an excellent place for newcomers to yoga to begin their practice. For example, beginning a student's practice on a chair may sometimes make them feel more successful while also improving their mobility so that they can later, if they so want, continue their practice on the mat.

In general, the following are some of the health benefits of yoga:

➤ The activation of the parasympathetic nervous system's soothing effects.

➤ Enhanced blood flow and circulation

➤ Bring down your blood pressure.

➤ Reduced levels of anxiety, hostility, irritation, and anger

➤ A more optimistic point of view

➤ Gains in muscular power

Research also reveals that chair yoga for seniors and chair yoga for beginners may be an intervention that is viable and safe to minimize the risk of falls, even for those in their 90s!

Additional advantages of sitting yoga for senior citizens include the following:

➤ Increases in both mobility and comfort for elderly patients suffering from osteoarthritis of the lower body

➤ A lessening of the ache

➤ Less fatigue

➤ Improvement in gait speed

# Why Chair Yoga?

Numerous studies have shown that practicing yoga may enhance a person's balance, strength, and stability. Unfortunately, as we age, we see a decline in our strength, balance, and overall stability. These three impairments are the primary contributors to the rise in the number of falls experienced by elderly citizens. One may not only halt the progression of the loss by engaging in yoga practice, but they can also buck the trend.

Yoga may be practiced by anyone of any age or physical ability. Practicing yoga can help you maintain strength and good health if you already have them. If you are dealing with health problems, whether temporary or chronic, a mild yoga practice may assist you in regaining some of the strength and flexibility you have lost as a result of your illness.

Traditional yoga, on the other hand, might be intimidating for those who are not as stable on their feet as they previously were, for people who wish to start slowly, or for people who feel more secure sitting down. So take a seat in the chair! You don't need to move from where you're sitting to get the advantages of yoga. Chair yoga not only has all of the benefits of regular yoga, such as relieving stress, pain, and fatigue, but it can also help with joint lubrication, balance, and arthritis. In addition, chair yoga is ideal for people with mobility issues or other conditions preventing them from performing traditional yoga poses.

One of the primary purposes of yoga is to improve and safeguard the spinal health of the practitioner. When we have bad posture, it disrupts the normal functioning of every component of our bodies. For example, a rounded back makes breathing difficult and limits blood flow. Regular yoga practice may improve your posture by extending and strengthening your spine. This will help you stand taller.

One further significant advantage of practicing yoga is the focus that is placed on the feet. Your feet are the primary determinant of your level of mobility. The majority of older adults, due to years of wear and tear, endure intermittent or occasionally chronic discomfort or numbness in their feet. This might result in reduced movement, which is a common contributing factor in accidents involving falling. The feet are actively engaged throughout a traditional yoga practice performed barefoot and without shoes. In every one of the exercises, I have positioned the stretching and strengthening of the feet to be the primary focus.

In my work, I have devised chair yoga routines that are simple to execute and appropriate for practitioners of varying degrees of fitness and experience. In this book, I discuss a good number of them. I expect that you will resolve to establish a habit of whatever new routine you choose to begin with. I believe that for a routine to become second nature, it must first and foremost be pleasurable to carry out before it can be considered successful.

Before I get into the routines, I want to tell you about some of my customers and friends to whom I have taught chair yoga, the effect it has had on their overall health, and how it has helped me better serve them. Most of my interactions with these individuals have taken the form of private one-on-one meetings. In this book, I outline different programs, and everything I do or have done with them is a component of one of those plans. Whenever I begin a new exercise, I almost always begin with the Beginner Program; nevertheless, in every one of these cases, I have progressed to the Intermediate level. Having a yoga instructor takes you through the different poses is beneficial. Because I have made a great effort to give the content in ways that are simple to comprehend, I would ask that you have confidence in anticipating outcomes. Because we care about maintaining everyone's privacy, the names have been altered.

# What are the Benefits of Chair Yoga?

It should be clear that chair yoga is an option for those with physical restrictions. It may also be ideal in specific circumstances when you have little space or time, such as while flying, sitting in a waiting room, or working in an office environment. Chair yoga, much like traditional yoga, is noted for its ability to improve one's strength, balance, and flexibility. This is because the motions are performed at a leisurely pace, enabling your body to stretch and hold certain positions comfortably and gently.

The strengthening of the neurological system that might result from practicing yoga's breathing exercises and relaxation methods can bring about a state of equilibrium in both the mind and the body. As is common knowledge, the relationship between the two is cooperative.

You'll experience feelings of serenity and relaxation directly from the breathing exercises that yoga encourages. The sympathetic nervous system (SNS) is the part of the nervous system responsible for producing reflex adjustments (like the fight or flight response). Diaphragmatic breathing helps move us into the parasympathetic response, the part of the nervous system responsible for the body's rest and digestion response when it is relaxed.

According to Organic Authority, "Yoga can effectively reduce the body's stress response by decreasing the production of cortisol," which occurs when the sympathetic nervous system is overworked. The physical postures, breathing techniques, and conscious relaxation strategies that assist activate the parasympathetic nervous system are what "the practice does this effectively by increasing the coordination between our minds and our bodies."

Consider chair yoga a physical rehabilitation or treatment, just as any other form of appropriate exercise may alleviate specific aches and pains or alleviate the physical symptoms of certain ailments. In addition, you probably already knew this, but doing yoga regularly may improve the quality of your sleep.

## Examples of Chair Yoga Poses

Instead of reading about the motions involved in chair yoga, it is ideal to see them being done and have hands-on experience with them. Look at the following illustration to see a variety of chair yoga positions.

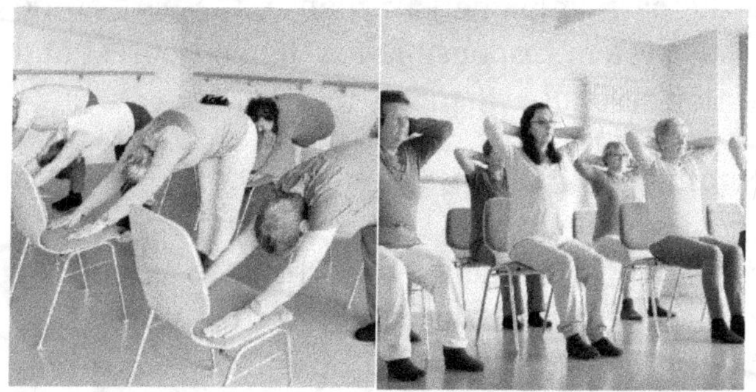

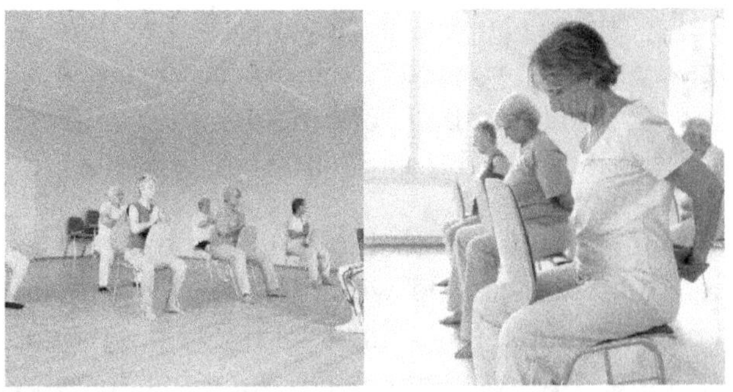

Maintain each posture for one to two full breaths, or for a longer time if you so want (profoundly breathing in through your nose and out, at a comfortable and relaxing pace.)

Keep in mind that there is no need to be haste while doing yoga. The important thing is to pay attention to your body and the things it requires. If you cannot find a comfortable stance, skip it or find a modification that will help you.

# Precautions

Consult your primary care provider before starting any fitness program, including chair yoga. Although chair yoga and the exercises in this book have the potential to enhance the effects of any current medical therapy, they are in no way meant to serve instead of conventional medical care.

I want you to improve your flexibility to continue to reach down to tie your shoes, safely get up and down from a chair, and have the strength and flexibility to get up and down off the floor if necessary. Chair yoga for seniors is designed to assist you in maintaining your independence for the most extended period feasible throughout your life.

Your pain-free range of motion is the range of motion that you can do without experiencing any kind of discomfort, including clicking or popping in your joints. Always keep your work inside these parameters. The practice of yoga shouldn't make you feel any worse. If something is uncomfortable, you can try a less strenuous variation of the posture, or you can ask your instructor for assistance in locating a modification that is appropriate for your body.

# Particular Concerns Regarding Health

If you have osteoporosis, you should move slowly and deliberately so that room may be created in your joints. Always employ a mild version of the twisting motion, and under no circumstances should you use your arms to push or drag yourself into a twisted posture.

Move from your hip joints and steer clear of rounding your back when bending forward. Imagine that you are moving forward using your chest rather than your forehead as the leading edge. Always try to avoid bouncing and impacting the object.

If you have high blood pressure, you should always keep your head higher than your heart. Move gently while being mindful of your surroundings.

When rising from a forward bend (for example, in a Sun Salutation), rise carefully to decrease the likelihood of feeling dizzy. Low blood pressure is one of the causes of dizziness.

# Equipment

## Clothing

Loose and comfortable clothing that allows you to move freely is ideal for equipment attire. If you want a standard waist, you can constantly adjust your belt a little bit, but pants with a flexible waist will provide you with the most freedom of movement. Also, check that you have adequate clothing to keep you warm.

## Yoga mat

Placing a yoga mat beneath your chair will prevent it from moving around while you move about on the floor. Also, the cushioning provided by a yoga mat will come in handy when you are in standing poses.

You may support your feet more comfortably using foam blocks, a bolster, or even a little stool if you choose. This will assist in guaranteeing that your feet are in a neutral position. You are free to prop your feet up on anything solid as it does not move. You could make do with a book (like an extensive dictionary) in a hurry, but a stack of books is not something I would advocate using since it would be precarious and may topple over.

## Safety

If you are using a wheelchair, you need to check that it is resting on a flat surface and that the brake is turned on.

Leaning against the chair: Any position in which you are leaning against the chair, such as standing forward fold, requires that you either push the chair up against a wall or ensure that all four legs are fully planted on a non-slip surface (like a yoga mat).

## General Tips

Find a comfortable chair to sit in, and if your feet cannot rest flat on the ground while you are seated, place a block, a bolster, or a stool beneath them.

Maintain a temperature in the room that is agreeable to the occupants. Take up as much space as possible in the chair, and loosen up your shoulders. Be happy and laugh often.

If at all feasible, practice yoga barefoot (taking our shoes and socks off gives us a chance to look at our feet). Toe socks are another option to consider if your feet tend to feel chilly rapidly.

Use socks that cover the toes and keep the feet warm while yet allowing the toes to move freely. Remember that wearing socks on smooth surfaces might make you quite slippery. When wearing socks, you must take extra precautions and stand on a yoga mat when practicing standing poses on smooth flooring.

# Get Yourself Warmed Up

Rub your hands to warm them up before beginning the tapping and self-massage method.

When you are supposed to tap on the places mentioned in the exercises, be sure to tap with a flat hand and stay away from the joints.

When massaging the places specified in the following exercises, use mild and moderate pressure around the joints and on sensitive areas such as your belly and face.

As a safety precaution, you should avoid tapping directly on the joints.

Only use little pressure while massaging someone.

The benefits include warming up the whole body

are:

➢ Increases the amount of blood that flows to the skin.

➢ Relaxes the muscles and loosens up the body.

➢ Boosts one's awareness of their body.

➢ Increases one's awareness as well as coordination.

# Warming different parts

## 1. Feet

Raise your right foot and rest it on your left knee while you do the same with your left foot. If you find that this causes discomfort, consider resting the foot lifted on a stool or bolster instead.

Take a close look at your foot; can you see any differences in color or texture?

Begin massaging your foot by beginning at the toes and working your way up to the top of your foot, then down to the heel, and finally back up to the toes.

Is it possible to clasp one hand and one foot together in the same manner that you would clasp your hands together and then interlace your fingers between your toes.

Do the same thing with your other foot.

## 2. Calves

A flat palm should be used to tap all parts of the calf gently.

Carry on for the length of about five breaths taken comfortably.

Repeat on the calf on the opposing side.

## 3. Knees

Rub the region surrounding the knee with massage oil.

Feel the calming warmth of your hands on your knee as you massage them gently together.

Carry on for the length of about five breaths taken comfortably.

Perform the previous step on the opposite knee.

## 4. Thighs

Tap and massage all thigh parts gently, including the rear of the leg.

Carry on for the length of about five breaths taken comfortably.

Repeat on the other side of your thigh.

## 5. Belly

Rub your stomach in a clockwise manner with very little pressure.

Carry on for the length of about five breaths taken comfortably.

## 6. Arms

Raise one arm and tap it with the hand not being raised. It is best to steer clear of tapping directly on your wrist, elbow, or shoulder joints.

Tap thoroughly on the inner and outer sides of your arm, forearm, and upper arm.

Rub your wrist, elbow, shoulder, and armpit with a light touch.

Carry on for the length of about five breaths taken comfortably.

Perform the previous step with the other arm.

## 7: The Head and the Neck

A massage that focuses on the head, neck, and face.

Perform a light massage on the front and back of your neck, face, and ears.

Carry on for a period equivalent to around ten–20 calm breaths.

## 8. Tapping on the chest

The bones on each side of your chest that protrude slightly outward immediately below the base of your neck are known as your collarbones.

Tap your fingernails softly on and around your collarbones and down along your sternum, also known as your breastbone, which is the flat bone in the middle of your chest.

Carry on for the length of about five breaths taken comfortably.

## 9. Rubbing the Heart

Rub the region above your heart, which is located on the left side of your chest, with the palm of your flat hand.

Carry on for the length of about five breaths taken comfortably.

# Getting Started

## Grounding

Take a seat in the chair, and place your hands on your lap or your knees. Imagine that you have never sat in a chair before and try to get a feeling of how it feels to have the weight of your body resting on the seat. How do your hips feel when they are resting on the chair? Gently move your body from side to side and front to back in a circular motion. Notice how the floor, bolster, stool, or blocks feel as you contact them with your feet. Put your shoulders at ease, and allow a natural flow to your breathing.

Raise your feet on a set of blocks or bolster if you find that your toes do not completely touch the ground when you are sitting.

# Meditation

Put either one or two minutes into the timer. Put your hands and shoulders down and relax.

Relax and try closing your eyes for a while. Bring your attention to the way you are breathing. Pay close attention to your breath as it passes through your nose, but don't make any conscious efforts to alter it in any way; instead, simply observe it.

Take note of whether it is relaxed or tense.

Check to see whether the duration of the inhalation and the exhale are the same.

Take note of the temperature of the air as it enters and exits your body and the air surrounding you.

# Exercises for the Breath

## Breathing through each nostril in turn

The practice of breathing through each nostril, in turn, is relaxing and helps to balance the two halves of the brain. You will be shutting each nostril one at a time with the thumb and finger of your right hand as you go through the motions of this exercise, which means that you will be alternating between breathing and exhaling via each of your nostrils. It is acceptable to use either hand depending on which one is most comfortable; the right hand has been used traditionally, but either hand may be utilized. I will explain the move while demonstrating it with my right hand.

When you seal each nostril, do it carefully, using just the right amount of pressure to prevent air from escaping through that particular nose. There shouldn't be much of a need to apply pressure here. While seated in a comfortable position, exhale entirely through both nostrils. While doing so, press your right thumb on your right nostril to close it, and breathe in through your left nostril.

Let go of your thumb and, while breathing through your right nostril, seal your left nostril with your right forefinger to prevent air from escaping.

Inhale through your right nostril while keeping

your left one closed for the time being.

When ready to exhale, remove your finger from your left nostril, place your right thumb over your right nostril, and exhale through your left nostril.

This concludes the first round. Beginning with one or two cycles, progressively increase the amount of time you spend breathing in this manner until you reach several minutes. After you have completed everything, sit back with your hands in your lap and breathe normally through both of your nostrils.

For alternate nostril breathing, the finger position that is shown in the three photographs that are just above this one is considered to be the more conventional one. Starting this posture may be more difficult if you have discomfort or stiffness in your hand or fingers. Test out both hand positions to find which one works best for you. Regardless of the posture in which you choose to practice this breathing method, you will still get some benefits from it.

If you want to give it a go, clench your right hand into a fist. Next, bring your thumb, middle finger, and ring finger into a straight line. Next, put the pointer and middle fingers of your other hand into the fleshy region at the base of your thumb.

Make sure that your hand's palm is always facing you. When you want to shut your right nostril, use your thumb, and when you want to close your left nostril, use the side of your ring finger. Continue doing breathing via your alternative nostrils as was instructed earlier.

# Three Core Components of Chair Yoga

My methodology for teaching chair yoga has evolved over the years, but it can be summed up in three words: community, compassion, and circulation. With this as a guide, you should be able to design a meaningful and valuable chair yoga practice applicable to various situations that individuals find themselves in. It seems to me that the most important thing I can do for my pupils is to encourage them to concentrate not on the things they cannot achieve but on the things they can. Not just on a physical level but also on a cerebral and emotional one; this has caused my pupils to feel a profound sense of connection.

# Community

Gather the horses (or chairs) around the community! Only in this class do we sit in a circle for the whole lesson. This represents completeness, community, and the bonds that bind us. Eye contact and the sense of being a part of something larger are two things that, in a population that is becoming older, I believe to be of the utmost importance. We note fewer people in our group, and if we become aware that someone is absent, we quickly wonder how they are doing and if they are okay. The first few minutes of class are dedicated to "mouth yoga," a euphemism for chatting and getting caught up. This is frequently the point at which I mentally alter my class to meet better the students where they currently are. My attention and worry are heartfelt. This establishes a tone that maintains the encouraging vibe for the whole of our time spent together as a group. It brightens our spirits and brings us closer together. In the end, yoga refers to a state of unity.

In addition, this is the only class in which I am both a student and an instructor during the program. I don't want to simply stand at the front of the class and lecture people much more experienced and knowledgeable than I am. Instead, I want to be a part of the energy generated by the practice. I don't change my body since many factors are specific to each person. I depend on my vocal signals and my example when I need to correct them. Because they are grouped in a circle, it is easier for them to reference each other and observe how the posture appears on other bodies that also have issues. This is not intended to be a comparison but rather an opportunity to appreciate each other's unique qualities and to celebrate and encourage one another.

# Compassion

I like to get the mood for self-compassion going right at the beginning of practice. My observations have led me to the conclusion that many women of our age consider "body shaming" to be an acceptable form of reference. In addition, I hear a lot of chatter about anti-aging treatments and how "it's all downhill from here." There is often a disconnection between them and their bodies. I approach the conversation with great compassion as I carefully navigate language, encouraging them to explore the possibility that becoming older is a luxury rather than a burden. It is often the first chance they have had to create space in their lives to love and care compassionately for their bodies. Compassion and appreciation make it possible for mental practice to provide the groundwork for physical practice. When we move with loving care toward our body rather than anxiety and condemnation, it makes a massive difference in the quality of the movement.

# Circulation

After the mood of the class has been established, it is time to start moving. Next, I look at ways to improve circulation throughout the whole body, particularly in the nooks and crannies that don't get much attention during our typical "sit, stand, walk" routines of the day. For example, it would help if you pretended that the chair was a prop and then utilized it. It enables many individuals to continue building postural strength while also accessing the full range of mobility that their bodies are capable of.

At the beginning of class, we warmly welcome our feet by spreading and elevating our toes, then putting them back down. Next, we relax our eyelids, elongate our spines, and focus on breathing. After establishing the ujjayi breath, I remind my students that they should never put their movement or posture ahead of their breath. In yoga, the focus should be on the breath rather than the poses. Of course, it is possible to sequence a class in an infinite number of different ways; nevertheless, the following is one arrangement that may facilitate circulation among a variety of pupils.

# ½ Sun Salutations from a Seated Position

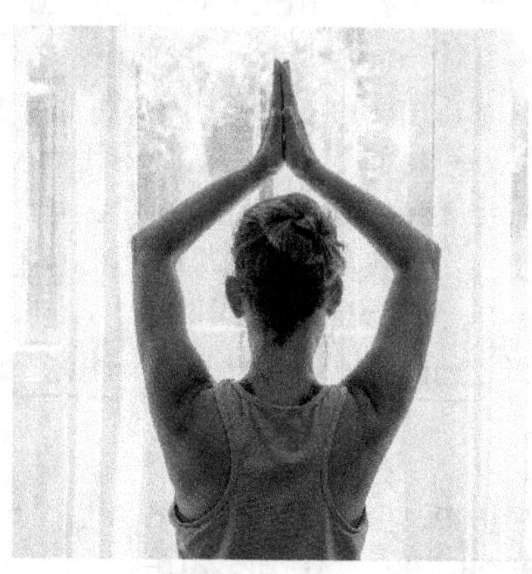

Every half of the breath-form moves us from one stance to the next, and it also starts to develop the link between the body and the mind. Perform three to five rounds of the following:

➢ Inhale: extending your arms over your head

➢ Exhale: Uttanasana

➢ Inhale and raise halfway

➢ Exhale: Uttanasana

➢ As you inhale, raise your arms over your head.

➢ Exhale, and bring your hands to your chest.

## Flexion and Extension (Better Known as Cat/Cow)

Inhale: Cow — Maintain as much of an upright posture as possible, rock onto your sitting bones, pull your shoulder blades together, and elevate your chin as you curl your sternum upward.

Cat: As you exhale, rock back behind your sitting bones and pull your sight towards your navel. Then, as you spread the back body-wide, could you bring it back towards your spine?

## Turn both to the right and left.

Maintain a lofty posture while bringing your knees and feet together. Bring your right hand to the outside of your left knee as you move it across your body. Put your left hand behind your back and stretch it to elevate the spine a bit higher.

While you exhale, twist your upper body to the left

while maintaining both sitting bones heavy and connected to the chair. Feel the length of your spine as you inhale, then twist your upper body as you exhale. Hold for between three and five breaths. Repeat on the other side, beginning with inhalation and ending with a release.

## Lateral bend The Right and the Left

Maintaining your current position in the chair, spread your feet about the width of a hip and press your sitting bones firmly onto the seat.

Take a breath in and raise both arms above. You should be able to side bend to the right without disconnecting your pelvis if you use your right hand to hold the left wrist. As you breathe gently and smoothly, make very few bounces to the right. There is no guarantee that the bounces will correspond to the breath. After staying here for three to five breaths, switch sides.

After the spinal column has been lubricated, it is time to focus on increasing circulation to the extremities.

## Shoulder Movements to the Front and Back

Put your fingers on the top of your arm bones, and as you inhale, shrug your shoulders and bring your elbows closer to your body. As you exhale, rotate your elbows out to the sides while simultaneously drawing your shoulder blades together and down. Repeat for three to five breaths. Alter your course for three to five breaths.

## Wrists

Put your fingers together in front of you and interlace them. Maintaining the position of the palms together, start rotating the hands in the same direction to make a circle. First, take it easy for two or three breaths, then pick up the pace for two or three additional breaths. Alternate holding hands with oneself by interlacing your fingers in a "weird way" instead of the traditional technique, and then continue to circle in the other direction.

## Hips/Ankles

Maintain a lofty sitting position and bring your right knee to your chest while holding it with your right hand. Start making circles with your right knee by rotating it to the right. After three to five revolutions, switch the circle's orientation. After that, stack your right thigh over your left like a sandwich. Start rotating your ankle in a clockwise circle for three breaths, then switch to rotating it in a counterclockwise circle. Garudasana is performed by maintaining the shape of the legs while beginning to press the outer shins towards each other and maybe tucking the right foot beneath the left calf (eagle pose). You may achieve this stance in a variety of different ways for a variety of reasons. Take advantage of this opportunity to give everyone the go-ahead to comfortably cross their legs and squeeze into whatever form they are capable of. Place your left arm on top of your right arm, and then wrap your hands over your outer armpits (they may only be able to hold opposite elbows instead of armpits). Raise your elbows till they are level with your shoulders. 3–5 deep breathes Continue in this manner on the left side, beginning with hip circles.

# Warrior 2 Seated

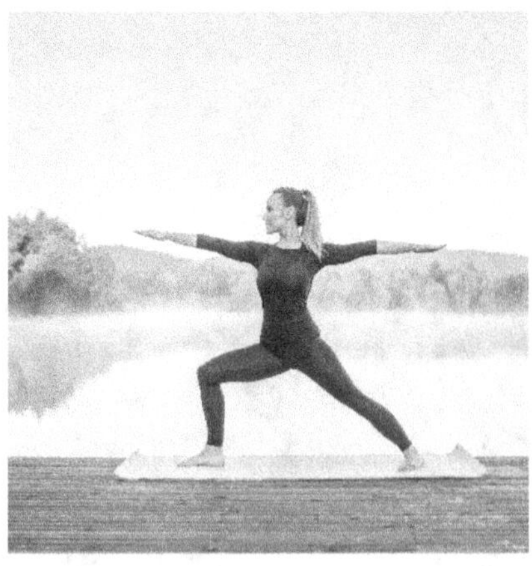

Make room for yourself on the right side of the chair. While sitting into your right thigh and sitting bone, turn your right knee and right foot to the right. Contracting your quadriceps will allow you to extend your left leg behind you. At the same time, turn your left foot out to the side. Spread your arms to the side, and rotate your upper body so that your shoulders and belly are towards the side. Count to five to seven before releasing. You might try doing the reverse warrior two and the side angle as a variant. It will be repeated on the left.

## Uttkatasana

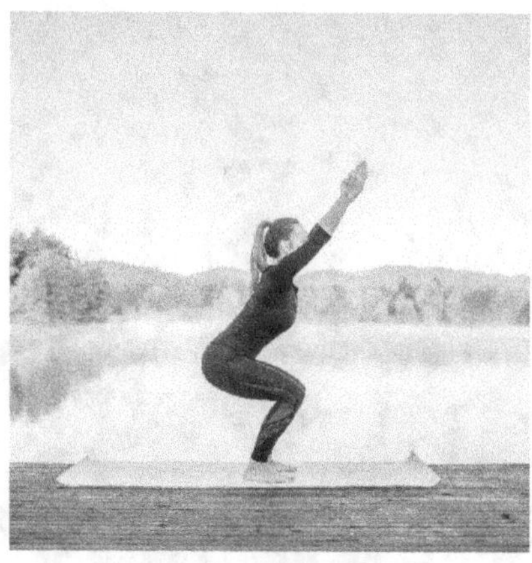

Place your feet about hip-distance apart from one another. While keeping your feet planted firmly on the ground, bring your heels back slightly below your knees and act as if you are spreading the floor with your feet. As you inhale, place your palms together in the Anjali mudra position and maintain your shoulders pulled back. Look ahead. Exhale, flex your hips ever-so-slightly, drive your heels to the floor, and raise your hips over the chair while keeping your chest and gaze facing forward (encourage students to use hands if necessary or just try to lift without coming out of the chair). Repeat this process three to five times. Inhale, then sit back down. The last one requires you to hover for three breaths, after which you should raise to a standking position on an inhale.

# The "Down Dog"

After reaching a standing position, instruct the children to spin the chair so that they may lay their hands on the chair's seat and step their feet back into the down dog position. Encourage a knee bend, a foot widening, and a posterior tilt higher than the head. In many cases, a "mini-workshop" is required to get them into the appropriate position. I first present a method that illustrates improper alignment, then describe the several health advantages associated with the down dog position. Pause for three to five breaths.

# Plank

When ready, you may go to the plank position from down dog. The plank pose is achieved by inhaling, while the down dog is attained by exhaling. Always on the table is the choice to remain in the dog. I advise bringing the inner armpits forward and releasing stiffness in the neck. When they are strong enough, you can also maintain the plank position or alternate between the plank and the dog position. Be active for five to ten breaths. Come to a finish in a down, dog, and then walk your feet back to your chair. Extend the back by doing a half lift. Raise yourself with a strong core and a flat back while bringing your hands to your hips and pointing your elbows toward the sky.

## Figure 4

Seat yourself in the chair after turning it around. To make a figure 4 form, flex the toes of your right foot and lay them on top of the knee of your left leg. Because many people's bodies need more support, this modification requires you to move your hands to the outside of the right shin and raise your body slightly. Be careful not to let your right foot become ill and sleep on the job. A good stretch will wake it up, and keeping the knee in this position will help preserve it. Next, hold three to five breaths while opening the right knee away from the right shoulder. It will be repeated on the left.

## Savasana

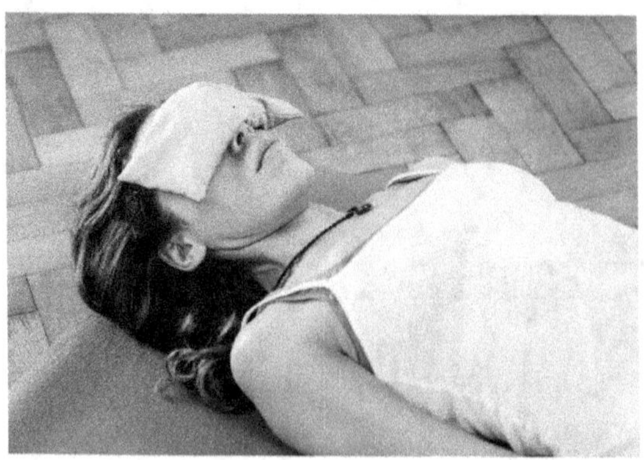

If you have a little additional time, you may integrate half sun salutations here; otherwise, you should find a comfortable resting posture while sitting back in the chair. Then, if the students can move up and down from the floor, I show them how to practice savasana with their legs on a chair. Continue with conscious breath for a further one to two minutes while receiving instruction, and then let everything go for two minutes.

# Warming up

I always start each workout with five minutes of light warm-ups to prepare my body. Our bodies are prepared to extend and stretch out during warm-ups, which is essential in reducing the risk of injury. The deep breathing exercises are an essential component of the warm-up. Obviously, as human beings, we never stop breathing. For us to carry it out, there is no need for us to contemplate it in any way. I'm referring to mindful breathing, in which you consciously direct your breathing to relax and make it easier for you to move about. According to many yoga instructors, the distinction between yoga and other forms of exercise is the deliberate inhalation and exhalation of air. I am aware that initially, this is a challenging idea to grasp. Still, I am confident that after you have established a level of familiarity with the routines in this book, you will comprehend the significance of the breath and welcome it into your practice. It is our source of strength, our means of relaxation, and our defense against danger.

# Mountain Pose

Position yourself in the beginning stage of the mountain pose by sitting up straight and tall on your chair, keeping your knees hip-width apart, and pointing your toes in a forward direction. Put your hands on your thighs while you do this. To improve your posture, roll your shoulders up and down your back, and draw your navel into your spine. When I speak to Mountain Pose from this point forward, you will understand that I intend for you to sit up tall in your chair with your shoulders up, back, and down, your knees hip distance apart, and your toes pointing straight ahead. Your hands should be resting on your thighs. Mountain Pose is the foundation of all chair yoga postures and serves as their final destination.

# The breath

Come to sit in Mountain Pose, which is the starting position.

Movement: Inhale slowly and steadily through your nose, and expel slowly and steadily through your mouth. This is one complete breath. Do not try to force your breath. Instead, it would help if you worked toward making the exhale duration equal to that of the inhale. For example, you may begin by counting to two on the inhale and then counting to two on the exhale to get you started. If you can make the pause between each inhale and exhale longer, for example, a count of three to four, then you should try to do so.

Repeatedly take four full breaths before continuing. Don't forget to go slow and steady.

The benefits of using this breathing style include reducing anxiety and calming the nervous system. In addition, it gets your muscles ready for action.

We often circle back to taking deep, cleansing breaths throughout our sessions. Have fun with them! They make you feel fantastic.

# Shoulder Shrugs

Mountain Pose is the starting position. Resume this pose.

Inhale as you pull both of your shoulders up to your ears and exhale as you return them to their neutral position at the beginning of the movement. Then, increase the amount of the lift.

Repeat this process a total of five times.

Advantages: Reduces the amount of strain on the neck and shoulders muscles.

Wrist Circles

As a starting position, assume the mountain pose, which involves sitting up straight. Place your belly button in line with your spine and draw the crown of your head up toward the ceiling as you sit.

Movement: Keep your elbows tight to your sides and reach your hands out in front of you while doing this action. Roll your hands around at the wrists while extending all of your fingers. Move your fingers around while simultaneously rolling your wrists.

Repetitions: Roll your wrists in one way, then switch and roll ten times in the other direction.

Advantages: Warms up the hands, including the wrists and fingers. Additionally reduces inflammation in the joints of the hand.

# Raise your arms above using both of them.

Take the position known as "Mountain Pose" to begin.

Movement: Raise both arms over your head while maintaining a calm and steady inhalation. Exhale slowly and steadily as you bring your arms back to the beginning position. During movement, make sure your shoulders remain relaxed. If raising your arms over your head makes you uncomfortable, you should instead lift them to a comfortable height.

Repetition: You should do this five times in total.

The benefits include increased arm strength as well as increased mobility in the shoulder joints.

## Knee Swings

Position yourself in Mountain Pose, with your shoulders back, and your tummy tucked up, and sit up tall.

Move your hands such that they are clasped beneath your right knee. Maintain a lofty and upright sitting position. While maintaining this position, kick your leg to the side in a back and forth motion. This is one of the few poses that we can do rather rapidly. If you cannot reach under your knee, you should lean back in the chair and kick out your right leg while swinging it back and forth at a reasonable pace. Again, if you cannot reach under your knee, you should continue with the next step.

The recommended number of repetitions for each leg is twenty.

Gains in mobility and range of motion in the knees are among the benefits.

# Exercises for the Ankles Using Both Legs

Mountain Pose is the starting position. Come into it.

Movement: While inhaling, elevate your spine and stretch both legs as far as you comfortably can. To attain this stance, ensure you are seated back in your chair. While trying to keep your legs completely straight, begin to spin your feet and ankles in a clockwise direction. Your feet and ankles are the only portions of your body that move when you sleep.

Perform ten revolutions in each direction to complete one repetition.

Benefits: Increases range of motion in the feet and ankles

Your pre-exercise warm-up is now finished. Your body is now prepared for an introductory yoga workout session that lasts fifteen minutes or twenty minutes if you choose the lengthier program. Always begin your workout with the same five-minute warm-up, no matter which regimen you choose. You should do the five-minute warm-up even if you have a few minutes to exercise. It beats the alternative of doing nothing at all by a significant margin. Side

# Neck Bend

Mountain Pose is the starting position. Come into it.

Movement: Take a deep breath in and sit up straight. As you let your breath out, bring the right ear down to the right shoulder. Check to see that your shoulders are loose and relaxed. To return your head to a neutral position, inhale. Now, take a deep breath to help you sit up straight, and then let out your breath as you bring your left ear to your left shoulder. Finally, take a deep breath to restore equilibrium to your brain. This is one of the sets.

Perform the set three times in a row as your repetitions.

The sides of the neck are stretched out, which is a benefit.

## Neck Turns

To return to the starting position, assume the mountain pose.

Movement: While inhaling, gradually rotate to the right with your head. As you let your breath out, come back to the center of your body very gently. While you are breathing in, gently move your head to the left. Return to the center while exhaling in a leisurely and even manner.

Perform the set three times in a row as your repetitions.

Benefits: Helps to restore mobility in the upper back and reduces stress in the neck and shoulders.

# Beginner Program

You have decided to begin your workout routine with the twenty-minute chair yoga program designed for beginners. Congratulations. I am delighted to hear that you want to give this a go. You will not despise this, as I had previously guaranteed to my customer Valerie.

I will go through the directions for the warm-up again here to save you the trouble of traveling back and forth in the book. First, however, please keep in mind my promise to you as the reader. Everything beyond this point is straightforward to read and comprehend.

## Mountain Pose

Position yourself in the beginning stage of the

mountain pose by sitting up straight and tall on your chair, keeping your knees hip-width apart, and pointing your toes in a forward direction. Put your hands on your thighs while you do this. To improve your posture, roll your shoulders up and down your back, and bring your navel into your spine.

## The breath

Come to sit in Mountain Pose, which is the starting position.

Movement: Inhale slowly and steadily through your nose, and expel slowly and steadily through your mouth. This is one complete breath. Do not try to force your breath. Instead, it would help if you worked toward making the exhale duration equal to that of the inhale. For example, you may begin by counting to two on the inhale and then counting to two on the exhale to get you started. If you can make the pause between each inhale and exhale longer, for example, a count of three to four, then you should try to do so.

Repeatedly take four full breaths before continuing. Don't forget to go slow and steady.

The benefits of using this breathing style include reducing anxiety and calming the nervous system. In addition, it gets your muscles ready for action.

## Side Neck Bend

Mountain Pose is the starting position. Come into it.

Movement: Take a deep breath in and sit up straight. As you let your breath out, bring the right ear down to the right shoulder. Check to see that your shoulders are loose and relaxed. To return your head to a neutral position, inhale. Now, take a deep breath to help you sit up straight, and then let out your breath as you bring your left ear to your left shoulder. Finally, take a deep breath to restore equilibrium to your brain. This is one of the sets.

Perform the set three times in a row as your repetitions.

The sides of the neck are stretched out, which is a benefit.

## Neck Turns

To return to the starting position, assume the mountain pose.

Movement: While inhaling, gradually rotate to the right with your head. As you let your breath out, come back to the center of your body very gently.

While you are breathing in, gently move your head to the left. Return to the center while exhaling in a leisurely and even manner.

Perform the set three times in a row as your repetitions.

Benefits: Helps to restore mobility in the upper back and reduces stress in the neck and shoulders.

## Shoulder Shrugs

Mountain Pose is the starting position. Resume this pose.

Inhale as you pull both of your shoulders up to your ears and exhale as you return them to their neutral position at the beginning of the movement. Then, increase the amount of the lift.

Repeat this process a total of five times.

Advantages: Reduces the amount of strain on the neck and shoulders muscles.

## Wrist Circles

Mountain Pose is the starting position. Sit up as tall

as you can. Place your belly button in line with your spine and draw the crown of your head up toward the ceiling as you sit.

Movement: Keep your elbows tight to your sides and reach your hands out in front of you while doing this action. Roll your hands around at the wrists while extending all of your fingers. Move your fingers around while simultaneously rolling your wrists.

Repetitions: Roll your wrists in one way, then switch and roll ten times in the other direction.

Advantages: Warms up the hands, including the wrists and fingers. Additionally reduces inflammation in the joints of the hand.

## Raise your arms above using both of them

Take the position known as "Mountain Pose" to begin.

Movement: Raise both arms over your head while maintaining a calm and steady inhalation. Exhale slowly and steadily as you bring your arms back to the beginning position. During movement, make sure your shoulders remain relaxed. If you find raising your arms above difficult, you should lift them to a more comfortable level.

Repetition: You will need to do this five times.

Advantages: Promotes shoulder joint flexibility and builds arms' strength.

## Knee Swings

Position yourself in Mountain Pose, with your shoulders back, and your tummy tucked up, and sit up tall.

Move your hands such that they are clasped beneath your right knee. Maintain an upright posture with a spine that is straight. While maintaining this position, kick your leg to the side in a back and forth motion. This is one of the few poses that we can do rather rapidly. If you cannot reach under your knee, you should lean back in the chair and kick out your right leg while swinging it back and forth at a reasonable pace. Again, if you cannot reach under your knee, you should continue with the next step.

The recommended number of repetitions for each leg is twenty.

Gains in mobility and range of motion in the knees are among the benefits.

## Complete a set of ankle circles with both legs

Mountain Pose is the starting position. Come into it.

Movement: While inhaling, elevate your spine and stretch both legs as far as you comfortably can. To attain this stance, ensure you are seated back in your chair. While trying to keep your legs completely straight, begin to spin your feet and ankles in a clockwise direction. Your feet and ankles are the only portions of your body that move when you sleep.

Perform ten revolutions in each direction to complete one repetition.

Benefits: Increases range of motion in the feet and ankles

Your pre-exercise warm-up is now finished. Let's stop for a moment and take three deep breaths together. Take a deep and steady breath through your nose, and then slowly and steadily let out your breath through your mouth.

## Shoulder Twists and Rolls

Mountain Pose is the starting position. Sit up as tall as you can.

Inhale as you raise your shoulders and back, and exhale as you return them to the beginning position. Movement: Inhale as you lift your shoulders up and back. Create as much of a seamless circle as possible with the movement by making it as fluid as possible. After you have completed five calm and steady circles, switch directions. As you inhale, push your shoulders toward your body as you lift them, and as you exhale, return your shoulders to their beginning position behind your neck. This course of action is inherently uncomfortable. You don't need to worry about it since you're already doing it right!

The exercise should be performed five times in each direction. The repetitions

Advantages: Increases flexibility and range of motion while opening the shoulder joints.

## Bending Forward While Maintaining a Straight Back

Position yourself in the starting position by sitting up straight in your chair and placing your hands on top of your thighs.

Movement: Bring your chin to your chest as you inhale and bend forward from the hips. Always remember to have a straight spine. It would help if you only went as far as possible while keeping a straight back. The hips are where the bend begins.

As you exhale, rise back to a standing position by placing your hands on your knees and utilizing them to propel you upward. Maintain your gaze on the path directly before you during the movement. Do not stare at your feet. This movement may not be significant, depending on how flexible your spine is. That is not in the least bit problematic. Keep in mind that the movement is quite sluggish!

To complete the repetitions, do each set five times.

Advantages: Increases flexibility in the back while simultaneously strengthening the muscles in the lower back

## Alternating Arm Raises

Mountain Pose is the starting position. Come into it.

Only do this action if it does not cause discomfort by lifting your right arm over your head while inhaling. If it isn't, you should elevate your arm as high as it is comfortable to go. Make an effort to maintain the straight position of your extended arm while keeping your shoulder relaxed. As you bring your arm closer to your body, exhale. Imagine that you are wading through water with one of your arms. You should gently move your arm. Turn the other cheek.

The repetitions are as follows: Repeat five times on each side.

Lubricating the shoulder joint is one of the benefits.

## Twist of the Torso with Arms Raise

Mountain Pose is the starting position. Sit up as tall as you can. Draw your belly in. Do it by rolling your shoulders forward, then back, and finally down your back.

Inhale as you pull both arms up as far as is comfortable while doing this movement. Shoulder blades are intense. Exhale. As you take a deep breath, rotate your upper body to the right. Keep your arms up, and keep your hips and legs pointing forward. You twist your head in the direction indicated by the movement. During the exhale, bring your focus back to the center. Maintain a raised arm position. Now, as you rotate your body to the left, inhale as you do so. Relax and come back to the middle. Place your hands in your lap when each round is complete.

Repeat each set of twists (a set includes both a right and a left twist). A set consists of both a right and a left twist.

The benefits include toning the waistline (love

handles) and promoting flexibility in the spine.

Let's halt here and make sure everyone has taken three deep breaths. First, take a deep and steady breath through your nose, and then slowly and steadily let out your breath through your mouth. You may find it helpful to close your eyes during the pauses we take for breathing. Again, it is beneficial for reducing stress and anxiety.

## Turning of the torso when the arms are extended out to the sides

Mountain Pose is the starting position, so get into it.

Extend your arms to the sides as you inhale as you do this movement. Exhale. While you are inhaling, gently rotate to your right. Your head moves in the same direction as your right arm when stretched. Exhale and come back to the center. Keep your arms at your sides. If you are using a mirror, check to verify that your shoulders are relaxed and your arms are at an equal length when extended. Take a deep breath in and rotate to your left. The left arm is responsible for transporting your head. Exhaling, bring your arms down to your knees and rest your hands until you return to the neutral position.

The repetitions are as follows: Perform each sequence of twists five times. Maintain an open posture with your arms throughout.

Advantages: Slims the waistline and builds strength in the arms.

## Lean to the side of your body while raising both arms.

Assume a good and lofty Mountain Pose sitting position as a starting position.

Movement: Take a deep breath as you lift both arms above and hold that position. Exhale. As you take your next breath, tilt your body to the right. Exhale as you lift your arms back up to neutral. At the same time, you are inhaling slowly and steadily, lean to your left side while keeping your arms up over your head. As you raise both arms above, let out an exhale. Check that your shoulders are not rounded forward toward your ears and that they are instead relaxed.

Perform five sets of repetitions. Throughout the workout, keep your arms up.

Benefits: Tones waistline.

## Single Arm and Leg Raises

Mountain Pose is the starting position. Come into it.

Movement: While lifting your right arm and right leg together at the same tempo, gradual and steady, inhale as you do so. As you gently drop your arm and leg, exhale as you do so.

Repetition: Do this five times, starting on the right side. To complete the left side, switch and repeat the previous five times.

Advantages: Builds muscle in the arms, legs, and core. Increases the level of coordination.

## Single-Leg Raises

Come into the starting position of Mountain Pose by coming to sit tall.

Movement: Inhale as you raise your right leg from its bent position and exhale as you lower it back to Mountain Pose. Inhale again as you lift your left leg from its bent position. Turn the other cheek. This is a gradual movement that is well managed.

The repetitions are as follows: repeat each side eight times.

Advantages: Increased mobility in the joint that controls the knee.

## Single Knee Raises

Mountain Pose is the starting position. Sit up as tall as you can.

Movement: Bring your right foot down to the

ground while gently lifting your right knee straight up off the ground. Raise your knee as far as you comfortably can.

Repetition: Perform this movement ten times on each side.

Advantages: It helps strengthen your quadriceps.

Let's stop once again, and every one of us should take three deep breaths. First, take a deep and steady breath through your nose, and then slowly and steadily let out your breath through your mouth.

## Point and Flex with a Single-Leg

Begin by taking a lofty position in your chair with your back completely straight.

Movement: While taking a deep breath, stretch your right leg in front of you straight. While maintaining this stance for your other leg, start pointing your right foot and flexing it. This may be done at a gradual pace or a fast one. In any case, you are giving your foot and ankle excellent exercise. Put your hands in whichever position is most at ease, whether down by your sides or in your lap. To the best of your ability, emphasize both the point and the flex. After you have completed the task, put your foot back on the ground and swap sides.

The number of repetitions is fifteen times on each side. Repeat.

In addition to strengthening the foot and ankle, this exercise stretches the shin and calf muscles.

## Single-Leg Ankle Circles

Mountain Pose is the starting position. Sit as tall as you can in your chair.

Movement: While inhaling, raise your right leg and begin to twist your foot clockwise. Continue to hold this position for the duration of the movement. The circles should be articulated slowly. Make sure they are as oversized and dramatic as you can make them. After around ten revolutions, you should change the direction you're going in. Maintain as much straightness in your elevated leg as you can. Swap out the legs.

Perform fifteen sets on each leg for the repetitions.

The benefits include increased mobility as well as strengthened ankles.

# Each of the Legs Points and Bends

Sit in the "Mountain Pose" as the starting position.

Movement: While taking a deep breath, stretch both legs in front of you straight. While maintaining this stance with your legs, proceed to point and flex each of your feet. This may be done at a gradual pace or a fast one. In any case, you are giving your feet and ankles excellent exercise. Put your hands in whichever position is most at ease, whether down by your sides or in your lap. To the best of your ability, emphasize both the point and the flex. When you are completed, place both feet flat on the ground.

Repeat this process a total of fifteen times.

In addition to strengthening the feet and ankles, this exercise stretches the shin and calf muscles.

## Heel Raises

The starting position consists of sitting tall and pointing both feet forward.

To do this movement, ensure that your toes are firmly placed on the floor, then proceed to elevate your heels. Maintain the lift in your heels while keeping your toes planted firmly on the ground. Exaggerate the heel lift with each repetition if you can do so comfortably.

Repeat this process a total of fifteen times.

Benefits: It stretches the muscles in your calves.

## Toe Raises

First, ensure that you sit straight and your feet point in front of you.

To perform this movement, ensure that your heels are firmly planted on the ground, and then begin lifting your toes. Maintain the lift on your toes while ensuring that your heels stay firmly on the floor. Exaggerate the lift each time, but only if you feel comfortable doing so.

Repeat this process a total of fifteen times.

The shins are stretched out, which is a benefit.

## Toe Squeeze

Sit in the "Mountain Pose" as the starting position.

Movement: Bring both legs forward and out to the sides while inhaling. Hold them in place while you squeeze your toes together as tightly as you can, then let go of the pressure and spread your toes as far apart as you can. Crunch once more, making sure that everything is as compact as possible! After that, let it loose and spread. Imagine that you can spread your toes so far apart that none of your toes are in contact with one another. In reality, this is just something to strive for in the future. After that, one or two of your toes will likely touch.

Repetition: Do this at least fifteen times in total. It's such a nice feeling!

The toes, feet, and ankles will all benefit from this stretch.

## Everything on the Table

Beginning Position: You have reached the final iteration of Mountain Pose for this chair yoga workout lasting twenty minutes. Make it a memorable experience. Maintain an elevated sitting position with your knees hip-distance apart and your toes pointing forward. Hold your stomach in toward your spine.

Movement: Raise your arms and legs slowly together as you inhale. Do this while keeping your back straight. Make an effort to keep all your limbs and your back as straight as possible while maintaining comfort. Exhale, then move your arms and legs back to the starting position as slowly as possible.

Repetition: Hold this pose a total of five times.

Benefits: Builds strength throughout the entire body.

# Deep Relaxation Pose

Position to Start: Lie on the seat, so the chair supports your back. Put your hands in a position of comfort on your lap, and then close your eyes.

Movement: Take nice, easy breaths and relax every muscle in your body. Permit yourself to relax all the muscles in your face, shoulders, legs, and feet.

Repetitions: Maintain this comfortable position for approximately five minutes while breathing in a natural and unforced manner.

Advantages: It makes it possible for your body to take in all of the positive effects of your yoga practice.

Congratulations! You have completed all of the steps in your routine. I hope that you are refreshed while also feeling completely at ease. I strongly encourage you to make it a priority to revisit this topic very shortly. Why not commit to doing it once every other day right now? The sooner you make chair yoga part of your routine, the sooner you will experience the myriad of life-improving benefits it offers.

And don't forget to drink some water. Your body needs it.

# Increasing the time

I am delighted to hear that you have decided to devote thirty minutes each day to the practice of chair yoga. We will be teaching you a few new positions and increasing the number of repetitions for the majority of the postures that you worked on throughout the first twenty minutes of the program. Always, we start with a five-minute warm-up to get ourselves ready.

Position yourself in the beginning stage of the mountain pose by sitting up straight and tall on your chair, keeping your knees hip-width apart, and pointing your toes in a forward direction. Put your hands on your thighs while you do this. To improve your posture, roll your shoulders up and down your back, and bring your navel into your spine.

# The breath

Come to sit in Mountain Pose, which is the starting position.

Movement: Inhale slowly and steadily through your nose, and expel slowly and steadily through your mouth. This is one complete breath. Do not try to force your breath. Instead, it would help if you worked toward making the exhale duration equal to that of the inhale. For example, you may begin by counting to two on the inhale and then counting to two on the exhale to get you started. If you can make the pause between each inhale and exhale longer, for example, a count of three to four, then you should try to do so.

Repeatedly take four full breaths before continuing. Don't forget to go slow and steady.

The benefits of using this breathing style include reducing anxiety and calming the nervous system. In addition, it gets your muscles ready for action.

## Side Neck Bend

Mountain Pose is the starting position. Come into it.

Movement: Take a deep breath in and sit up straight. As you let your breath out, bring the right ear down to the right shoulder. Check to see that your shoulders are loose and relaxed. Next, take a deep breath to restore equilibrium to your brain. Now, take a deep breath to help you sit up straight, and then let out your breath as you bring your left ear to your left shoulder. Again, take a deep breath to restore equilibrium to your brain. This is one of the sets.

Perform the set three times in a row as your repetitions.

The sides of the neck are stretched out, which is a benefit.

## Neck Turns

To return to the starting position, assume the mountain pose.

Movement: While inhaling, gradually rotate to the right with your head. As you let your breath out, come back to the center of your body very gently. While you are breathing in, gently move your head to the left. Return to the center while exhaling in a leisurely and even manner.

Perform the set three times in a row as your repetitions.

Benefits: Helps to restore mobility in the upper back and reduces stress in the neck and shoulders.

## Shoulder Shrugs

Mountain Pose is the starting position. Resume this pose.

Inhale as you pull both of your shoulders up to your ears and exhale as you return them to their neutral position at the beginning of the movement. Then, increase the amount of the lift.

Repeat this process a total of five times.

Advantages: Reduces the amount of strain on the neck and shoulders muscles.

## Rings on the Wrists

Mountain Pose is the starting position. Sit up as tall as you can. Place your belly button in line with your spine and draw the crown of your head up toward the ceiling as you sit.

Movement: Keep your elbows tight to your sides and reach your hands out in front of you while doing this action. Roll your hands around at the wrists while extending all of your fingers. Move your fingers around while simultaneously rolling your wrists.

Repetitions: Roll your wrists in one way, then switch and roll ten times in the other direction.

Advantages: Warms up the hands, including the

wrists and fingers. Additionally reduces inflammation in the joints of the hand.

## Raise your arms above using both of them

Take the position known as "Mountain Pose" to begin.

Movement: Raise both arms over your head while maintaining a calm and steady inhalation. Exhale slowly and steadily as you bring your arms back to the beginning position. During movement, make sure your shoulders remain relaxed. If you find raising your arms above difficult, you should lift them to a more comfortable level.

Repetition: You will need to do this five times.

Advantages: Promotes shoulder joint flexibility and builds arms' strength.

## Knee Swings

Position yourself in Mountain Pose, with your shoulders back, and your tummy tucked up, and sit up tall.

Move your hands such that they are clasped beneath your right knee. Maintain an upright posture with a spine that is straight. While maintaining this position, kick your leg to the side in a back and forth motion. This is one of the few poses that we can do rather rapidly. If you cannot reach under your knee, you should lean back in the chair and kick out your right leg while swinging it back and forth at a reasonable pace. Again, if you cannot reach under your knee, you should continue with the next step.

The recommended number of repetitions for each leg is twenty.

Gains in mobility and range of motion in the knees are among the benefits.

## Complete a set of ankle circles with both legs

Mountain Pose is the starting position. Come into it.

Movement: While inhaling, elevate your spine and stretch both legs as far as you comfortably can. To attain this stance, ensure you are seated back in your chair. While trying to keep your legs completely straight, begin to spin your feet and ankles in a clockwise direction. Your feet and ankles are the only portions of your body that move when you sleep.

Perform ten revolutions in each direction to complete one repetition.

Advantages: Increases range of motion in the feet and ankles.

Our pregame warm-up is now over. Let's begin!

## Rolls with the Hands on the Shoulders

Mountain Pose is the starting position, so come into that.

Movement: With your hands resting on top of your shoulders, move your shoulders in huge circles while guiding them with your elbows. Maintain a relaxed breathing pattern as you move. Alter the direction in which your circles are going.

Repeat steps one through eight times in each direction.

The benefits include relaxing the stiffness in your neck and warming up your upper back.

## Shoulder Twists and Rolls

Mountain Pose is the starting position. Sit up as tall as you can.

Inhale as you raise your shoulders and back, and

exhale as you return them to the beginning position. Movement: Inhale as you lift your shoulders up and back. Create as much of a seamless circle as possible with the movement by making it as fluid as possible. After you have completed five calm and steady circles, switch directions. As you inhale, push your shoulders toward your body as you lift them, and as you exhale, return your shoulders to their beginning position behind your neck. This course of action is inherently uncomfortable. You don't need to worry about it since you're already doing it right!

The exercise should be performed five times in each direction. The repetitions

Advantages: Increases flexibility and range of motion while opening the shoulder joints.

## Bending Forward While Maintaining a Straight Back

Position yourself in the starting position by sitting up straight in your chair and placing your hands on top of your thighs.

Movement: Bring your chin to your chest as you inhale and bend forward from the hips. Always remember to have a straight spine. You should only go as far as possible while keeping a straight back. The hips are where the bend begins. As you exhale, rise back to a standing position by placing your hands on your knees and utilizing them to propel you upward. Maintain your gaze on the path directly before you during the movement. Do not stare at your feet. This movement may not be significant, depending on how flexible your spine is. That is not in the least bit problematic. Keep in mind that the movement is quite sluggish!

To complete the repetitions, do each set five times.

Advantages: Increases flexibility in the back while simultaneously strengthening the muscles in the lower back

## Alternating Arm Raises

Mountain Pose is the starting position. Come into it.

Only do this action if it does not cause discomfort by lifting your right arm over your head while inhaling. If it isn't, you should elevate your arm as high as it is comfortable to go. Make an effort to maintain the straight position of your extended arm while keeping your shoulder relaxed. As you bring your arm closer to your body, exhale. Turn the other cheek.

The repetitions are as follows: repeat each side eight times.

Lubricating the shoulder joint is one of the benefits.

## Extend(ing) Their Arms Palm Rotation

Mountain Pose is the starting position, with the shoulders pulled back and the spine in a neutral position.

Movement: Extend both arms straight to the sides of your body with your palms facing upward. Maintain an extended stance with your arms while relaxing your shoulders. You should start by turning your hands so that they are facing down and then back to the up position. Your hands are the only things that move. Maintain a regular breathing pattern throughout.

Repeat this sequence five times and then come back to the mountain pose. After performing an inhalation and an exhale, you will repeat the exercise ten times.

The benefits include building strength in the arms and warming up the shoulders.

## Extend(ing) Their Arms Hand Squeeze

Sit up tall in Mountain Pose, which is the starting position.

Move: Extend both arms in a straight line out to the sides of your body. It would help if you made a tight fist with your fingers while taking a calm, steady breath and then let out your breath while stretching out your fingers exaggeratedly.

The repetitions are as follows: Perform each set ten times. Bring your body back into Mountain Pose. Perform the exercise for a total of ten sets.

The benefits include strengthening and stretching the hands and fingers. Carpal tunnel syndrome patients will benefit greatly from this activity.

## Twist of the Torso with Arms Raise

Mountain Pose is the starting position. Sit up as tall as you can. Draw your belly in. Do it by rolling your shoulders forward, then back, and finally down your back.

Inhale as you pull both arms up as far as is comfortable while doing this movement. Shoulder blades are intense. Exhale. As you take a deep breath, rotate your upper body to the right. Keep your arms up, and keep your hips and legs pointing forward. You twist your head in the direction indicated by the movement. During the exhale, bring your focus back to the center. Maintain a raised arm position. Now, as you rotate your body to the left, inhale as you do so. Relax and come back to the middle. Place your hands in your lap when each round is complete.

To complete the repetitions, you will do each set of twists (a set consisting of a good twist and a left twist) eight times.

The benefits include toning the waistline (love handles) and promoting flexibility in the spine.

Let's halt here and make sure everyone has taken three deep breaths. First, take a deep and steady breath through your nose, and then slowly and steadily let out your breath through your mouth. You may find it helpful to close your eyes during the pauses we take for breathing. Again, it is beneficial for reducing stress and anxiety.

## Turning of the torso when the arms are extended out to the sides

Mountain Pose is the starting position, so get into it.

Extend your arms to the sides as you inhale as you do this movement. Exhale. While you are inhaling, gently rotate to your right. Your head moves in the same direction as your right arm when stretched. Exhale and come back to the center. Keep your arms at your sides. If you are using a mirror, check to verify that your shoulders are relaxed and your arms are at an equal length when extended. Take a deep breath in and rotate to your left. The left arm is responsible for transporting your head. Exhaling, bring your arms down to your knees and rest your hands until you return to the neutral position.

The repetitions are as follows: Perform each set eight times.

Advantages: Slims the waistline and builds strength in the arms.

## Back Bend

Mountain Pose is the starting position. Come into it.

Move your hands, so they are resting on your legs with your palms facing down. Inhale slowly and steadily as you elevate your chest, gently arch your back, open your shoulders, and look upward toward the ceiling while you do so. While you are exhaling, bring your eyes down to the ground as you gently lower your head, round your back, and your shoulders. Now you should go back to neutral. Let's go back and try it again. When you inhale, ensure that you simultaneously lift your chest, arch your back, open your shoulders, and look up. Then, when you exhale, ensure you are doing the same thing. Some practice may be required, but the results will be well worth it.

Repeat this stance five times over your whole practice.

Advantages: It helps to warm up the lumbar and thoracic spine (upper and lower back). Encourages a healthy posture.

## Lean to the side of your body while raising both arms

Assume a good and lofty Mountain Pose sitting position as a starting position.

Movement: Take a deep breath as you lift both arms above and hold that position. Exhale. As you take your next breath, tilt your body to the right. As you bring your arms back to the neutral position, exhale as you do so. At the same time, you are inhaling slowly and steadily, lean to your left side while keeping your arms up over your head. As you raise both arms above, let out an exhale. Check that your shoulders are not rounded forward toward your ears and that they are instead relaxed.

Perform a total of eight sets of repetitions. Throughout the workout, keep your arms up. Hold the posture on each side for the last repetition, and breathe fully before releasing the pose. Relax into the posture, then go back to the starting position.

Benefits: Tones waistline.

## Twist in the Chair

Position to begin: Sit up straight with your feet about hip-width apart.

Movement: Starting in an upright position, slowly rotate your upper body to the right and place your right hand on the top of the chair's back. Position your left hand such that it is on the outside of your right knee. Check that the front of both of your knees is facing the same direction. Lift your spine as you inhale, and then exhale as you gently twist to the right as you continue to twist. Get back to the neutral position. It takes considerable work to achieve this stance. Make sure that your lower body does not move at all!

The repetitions are as follows: Repeat five times on each side.

Benefits include massaging the internal organs and tightening the abdominal muscles.

## Single Arm and Leg Raises

Mountain Pose is the starting position. Come into it.

Movement: While lifting your right arm and right leg together at the same tempo, gradual and steady, inhale as you do so. As you gently drop your arm and leg, exhale as you do so.

Repetition: Perform this movement ten times on each side.

Advantages: Builds muscle in the arms, legs, and core. Increases the level of coordination.

Single-Leg Raises

Come into the starting position of Mountain Pose by coming to sit tall.

Movement: Inhale as you raise your right leg from its bent position and exhale as you lower it back to Mountain Pose. Inhale again as you lift your left leg from its bent position. Turn the other cheek. This is a gradual movement that is well managed.

Repetition: Perform this movement ten times on each side.

Advantages: Increased mobility in the joint that controls the knee.

## Single Knee Raises

Mountain Pose is the starting position. Sit up as tall as you can.

Movement: Bring your right foot down to the ground while gently lifting your right knee straight up off the ground. Raise your knee as far as you comfortably can.

Repetition: Perform this movement ten times on

each side.

Advantages: It helps strengthen your quadriceps.

Let's stop once again, and everyone should take three deep breaths. First, take a deep and steady breath through your nose, and then slowly and steadily let out your breath through your mouth.

## Point and Flex with a Single-Leg

Begin by taking a lofty position in your chair with your back completely straight.

Movement: While taking a deep breath, stretch your right leg in front of you straight. While maintaining this stance for your other leg, start pointing your right foot and flexing it. This may be done at a gradual pace or a fast one. In any case, you are giving your foot and ankle excellent exercise. Next, put your hands in whichever position is most at ease for you, whether down by your sides or in your lap. To the best of your ability, emphasize both the point and the flex. After you have completed the task, put your foot back on the ground and swap sides.

The number of repetitions is fifteen times on each side. Repeat.

In addition to strengthening the foot and ankle, this

exercise stretches the shin and calf muscles.

## Single-Leg Ankle Circles

Mountain Pose is the starting position. Sit as tall as you can in your chair.

Movement: While inhaling, raise your right leg and begin to twist your foot clockwise. Continue to hold this position for the duration of the movement. The circles should be articulated slowly. Make sure they are as oversized and dramatic as you can make them. After around ten revolutions, you should change the direction you're going in. Maintain as much straightness in your elevated leg as you can. Swap out the legs.

Ten sets on each side constitute one repetition.

The benefits include increased mobility as well as strengthened ankles.

## Each of the Legs Points and Bends

Sit in the "Mountain Pose" as the starting position.

Movement: While taking a deep breath, stretch

both legs in front of you straight. While maintaining this stance with your legs, proceed to point and flex each of your feet. This may be done at a gradual pace or a fast one. In any case, you are giving your feet and ankles excellent exercise. Put your hands in whichever position is most at ease, whether down by your sides or in your lap. To the best of your ability, emphasize both the point and the flex. When you are completed, place both feet flat on the ground.

Repeat this process a total of fifteen times.

In addition to strengthening the feet and ankles, this exercise stretches the shin and calf muscles.

## Heel Raises

The starting position consists of sitting tall and pointing both feet forward.

To do this movement, ensure that your toes are firmly placed on the floor, then proceed to elevate your heels. Maintain the lift in your heels while keeping your toes planted firmly on the ground. Exaggerate the heel lift with each repetition if you can do so comfortably.

Repeat this process a total of fifteen times.

Benefits: It stretches the muscles in your calves.

## Toe Raises

First, ensure that you sit straight and your feet point in front of you.

To do this movement, ensure that your heels are securely placed on the ground and elevate your toes. Maintain the lift on your toes while ensuring that your heels stay firmly on the floor. Exaggerate the lift each time, but only if you feel comfortable doing so.

Repeat this process a total of fifteen times.

The shins are stretched out, which is a benefit.

## Toe Squeeze

Sit in the "Mountain Pose" as the starting position.

Movement: Bring both legs forward and out to the sides while inhaling. Hold them in place as you pinch your toes together as firmly as you can, then let go of the pressure and spread your toes as far apart as you can. Crunch once more, making sure that everything is as compact as possible! After that, let it loose and spread. Imagine that you can stretch your toes so far apart that none of your toes are in contact with one another. In reality, this is only something to strive toward in the future. One or two of your toes will probably contact.

Repetition: Do this at least fifteen times in total. It's such a nice feeling!

The toes, feet, and ankles will all benefit from this stretch.

## Everything on the Table

Beginning Position: You have reached the end of your mountain pose sequence for your chair yoga practice that lasted thirty minutes. Make it a memorable experience. Maintain an elevated sitting position with your knees hip apart and your toes pointing forward. Hold your stomach in toward your spine.

Movement: Raise your arms and legs gently together as you inhale. Do this while keeping your back straight. Make an effort to keep all your limbs and your back as straight as possible while maintaining comfort. Exhale, then move your arms and legs back to the beginning position as gently as possible.

Repetition: Hold this stance a total of eight times.

Benefits: Builds strength throughout the whole body.

## Position for Deep Relaxation

Position to Start: Lie on the seat, so the chair supports your back. Put your hands in a position of comfort on your lap, and then shut your eyes.

Movement: Take nice, easy breaths and relax every muscle in your body. Permit yourself to relax all the muscles in your face, shoulders, legs, and feet.

Repetitions: Maintain this comfortable position for approximately five minutes while breathing in a natural and unforced manner.

Advantages: It makes it possible for your body to take in all of the positive effects of your yoga practice.

You have completed your tasks for the day! Take a sip of water and savor the feeling of accomplishment that comes from knowing you're taking care of yourself.

# Intermediate Level of Practice

I want to extend my warmest greetings to you as you enter this new level of commitment, whether you are moving up to the intermediate level for the first time or have advanced to it after completing the beginning program. In this routine, we are going to make the movements more challenging, but we are going to do it in a manner that is both safe and realistic. The only new equipment you will need is two dumbbells weighing two pounds each. After a few months of training three to five times per week, most of my students can go from working with weights weighing two pounds to working with weights weighing three or even four pounds. Put this information aside for further review at a later time.

I'd like to draw your attention to a couple of things on our getting started checklist, which are as follows:

• Put some water in your system.

• Dress in a relaxed manner.

• Have some of your favorite music prepared and ready to play.

• Position your chair in an area that is free of clutter.

• When walking on any kind of floor surface, either go barefoot or wear shoes with rubber soles. When walking on the carpet, just wear socks.

• Make room for this book on your music stand by placing it there. Positioning the book so that it is at eye level is quite helpful.

• Put the dumbbells where they are easily accessible.

We are prepared to get started! Let's get the warm-up started.

Position yourself in the beginning stage of the mountain pose by sitting up straight and tall on your chair, keeping your knees hip-width apart, and pointing your toes in a forward direction. Put your hands on your thighs while you do this. To improve your posture, roll your shoulders up and down your back, and bring your navel into your spine.

# The breath

Come to sit in Mountain Pose, which is the starting position.

Movement: Inhale slowly and steadily through your nose, and expel slowly and steadily through your mouth. This is one complete breath. Do not try to force your breath. Instead, you should work toward making the exhale duration equal to that of the inhale. For example, you may begin by counting to two on the inhale and then counting to two on the exhale to get you started. If you can make the pause between each inhale and exhale longer, for example, a count of three to four, then you should try to do so.

Repeatedly take four full breaths before continuing. Don't forget to go slow and steady.

The benefits of using this breathing style include reducing anxiety and calming the nervous system. In addition, it gets your muscles ready for action.

## Side Neck Bend

Mountain Pose is the starting position. Come into it.

Movement: Take a deep breath in and sit up straight. As you let your breath out, bring the right ear down to the right shoulder. Check to see that your shoulders are loose and relaxed. Take a deep breath to restore equilibrium to your brain. Now, take a deep breath to help you sit up straight, and then let out your breath as you bring your left ear to your left shoulder. Again, take a deep breath to restore equilibrium to your brain. This is one of the sets.

Perform the set three times in a row as your repetitions.

The sides of the neck are stretched out, which is a benefit.

## Neck Turns

To return to the starting position, assume the mountain pose.

Movement: While inhaling, gradually rotate to the right with your head. As you let your breath out, come back to the center of your body very gently. While you are breathing in, gently move your head to the left. Return to the center while exhaling in a leisurely and even manner.

Perform the set three times in a row as your repetitions.

Benefits: Helps to restore mobility in the upper back and reduces stress in the neck and shoulders.

## Shoulder Shrugs

Mountain Pose is the starting position. Resume this pose.

Inhale as you pull both of your shoulders up to your ears and exhale as you return them to their neutral position at the beginning of the movement. Then, increase the amount of the lift.

Repeat this process a total of five times.

Advantages: Reduces the amount of strain on the neck and shoulders muscles.

## Rings on the Wrists

Mountain Pose is the starting position. Sit up as tall as you can. Place your belly button in line with your spine and draw the crown of your head up toward the ceiling as you sit.

Movement: Keep your elbows tight to your sides and reach your hands out in front of you while doing this action. Roll your hands around at the wrists while extending all of your fingers. Move your fingers around while simultaneously rolling your wrists.

Repetitions: Roll your wrists in one way, then switch and roll ten times in the other direction.

Advantages: Warms up the hands, including the wrists and fingers. Additionally reduces inflammation in the joints of the hand.

## Raise your arms above using both of them

Take the position known as "Mountain Pose" to begin.

Movement: Raise both arms over your head while maintaining a calm and steady inhalation. Exhale slowly and steadily as you bring your arms back to the beginning position. During movement, make sure your shoulders remain relaxed. If you find raising your arms above difficult, you should lift them to a more comfortable level.

Repetition: You will need to do this five times.

Advantages: Promotes shoulder joint flexibility and builds arms' strength.

## Knee Swings

Position yourself in Mountain Pose, with your shoulders back, and your tummy tucked up, and sit up tall.

Move your hands such that they are clasped beneath your right knee. Maintain an upright posture with a spine that is straight. While maintaining this position, kick your leg to the side in a back and forth motion. This is one of the few poses that we can do rather rapidly. If you cannot reach under your knee, you should lean back in the chair and kick out your right leg while swinging it back and forth at a reasonable pace. Again, if you cannot reach under your knee, you should continue with the next step.

The recommended number of repetitions for each leg is twenty.

Gains in mobility and range of motion in the knees are among the benefits.

## Complete a set of ankle circles with both legs

Mountain Pose is the starting position. Come into it.

Movement: While inhaling, elevate your spine and stretch both legs as far as you comfortably can. To attain this stance, ensure you are seated back in your chair. While trying to keep your legs completely straight, begin to spin your feet and ankles in a clockwise direction. Your feet and ankles are the only portions of your body that move when you sleep.

Perform ten revolutions in each direction to complete one repetition.

Benefits: Increases range of motion in the feet and ankles

The warm-up portion of our workout is now complete. Let's get started with our yoga session on the chair.

## Rolls with the Hands on the Shoulders

Mountain Pose is the starting position, so come into that.

Movement: With your hands resting on top of your shoulders, move your shoulders in huge circles while guiding them with your elbows. Maintain a relaxed breathing pattern as you move. Alter the direction in which your circles are going.

Repeat steps one through eight times in each direction.

The benefits include relaxing the stiffness in your neck and warming up your upper back.

## Shoulder Twists and Rolls

Mountain Pose is the starting position. Sit up as tall as you can.

Inhale as you raise your shoulders and back, and exhale as you return them to the beginning position. Movement: Inhale as you lift your shoulders up and back. Create as much of a seamless circle as possible with the movement by making it as fluid as possible. After you have completed five calm and steady circles, switch directions. As you inhale, push your shoulders toward your body as you lift them, and as you exhale, return your shoulders to their beginning position behind your neck. This course of action is inherently uncomfortable. You don't need to worry about it since you're already doing it right!

The exercise should be performed eight times in each direction. The repetitions

Advantages: Increases flexibility and range of motion while opening the shoulder joints.

# Bending Forward While Maintaining a Straight Back

Position yourself in the starting position by sitting up straight in your chair and placing your hands on top of your thighs.

Movement: Bring your chin to your chest as you inhale and bend forward from the hips. Always remember to have a straight spine. You should only go as far as possible while keeping a straight back. The hips are where the bend begins. As you exhale, rise back to a standing position by placing your hands on your knees and utilizing them to propel you upward. Maintain your gaze on the path directly before you during the movement. Do not stare at your feet. This movement may not be very significant, depending on how flexible your spine is. That is not in the least bit problematic. Keep in mind that the movement is quite sluggish!

Repeat this process a total of eight times. Hold the bent posture for the eighth repetition while taking one complete breath that consists of a slow, steady intake and a slow, steady exhale. This is one whole breath. Get back to being neutral.

Advantages: Increases flexibility in the back while simultaneously strengthening the muscles in the lower back

# Arm Raises interspersed with Weighted Exercises

Come into Mountain Pose while holding the two-pound weights in each hand and letting them rest on your thighs. This is your starting position.

Only do this action if it does not cause discomfort by lifting your right arm over your head while inhaling. If it isn't, you should elevate your arm as high as it is comfortable to go. Make an effort to maintain the straight position of your extended arm while keeping your shoulder relaxed. As you bring your arm closer to your body, exhale. Turn the other cheek.

Repetition: You will need to do this six times on each side. On the last repetition on each side, hold the posture and be sure to take a complete breath before moving on. Relax into the posture, then go back to the starting position. Throughout the workout, you are holding the weights in both hands.

Advantages include arm strengthening as well as lubrication of the shoulder joint.

## Rotation of the trunk while holding weights in extended arms

Mountain Pose is the starting position; hold

weights in both hands and assume this position.

Movement: While holding a weight in each hand, begin by extending your arms to the sides of your body as you inhale. Exhale. While you are inhaling, gently rotate to your right. Your head moves in the same direction as your right arm when stretched. Exhale and come back to the center. Keep your arms at your sides. If you are using a mirror, you should ensure that your shoulders are relaxed and that your arms are at shoulder level as you stretch them. Take a deep breath in and rotate to your left. The left arm is responsible for transporting your head. Bring your arms down until resting on your legs, and then return to the neutral position.

The repetitions are as follows: Perform each set eight times. While holding the position for the last repetition on either side, inhale fully before releasing it. Relax into the posture, then go back to the starting position.

Advantages: Slims the waistline and builds strength in the arms.

Let's stop for a moment and take three deep breaths together. First, take a deep and steady breath through your nose, and then slowly and steadily let out your breath through your mouth.

# Exercise for the Side of the Body Using Weights

As a starting position, assume a good and lofty Mountain Pose are sitting position. Next, place the weights in each of your hands on your thighs.

Inhale as you pull both arms up and maintain this position while holding weights in both hands. Movement: Exhale. As you take your next breath, tilt your body to the right. As you bring your arms back to the neutral position, exhale as you do so. At the same time, you are inhaling slowly and steadily, lean to your left side while keeping your arms up over your head. As you bring both arms back up to the overhead position, exhale.

Perform a total of eight sets of repetitions. The arms remain up throughout. Hold the posture for the last repetition on each side, and breathe fully before releasing the pose. Relax into the posture, then go back to the starting position.

Benefits: Tones waistline.

# Bicep Curls with Weights, Performing Alternating Arms

Come to a sitting position in Mountain Pose with the weights in your hands. This is your starting position.

Movement: Bring your arms down to your sides and rest them there. Maintain a position in which your elbows are firmly affixed to the sides of your body. Your right arm should be bent up gently as you inhale, and you should exhale as it is lowered back to the starting position. Take a deep breath as you raise your left arm, and then let out as you lower it back to the starting position. Throughout the action, your elbows will remain firmly planted at your sides.

The repetitions are as follows: repeat each side eight times. Then, after taking a hiatus, continue t

Biceps muscle may be built up with regular use of this product.

## Raise your arms and legs individually using weights.

Mountain Pose is the starting position. Bring some weights onto your lap and come into Mountain Pose.

Movement: Take a deep breath as you raise your right leg and right arm (the weight should be in your hand). The arm and the leg should be held in the straightest position possible. As you bring them down, exhale as you do so.

Repetition: You will need to do this six times on each side. On the last repetition of each side, pause in the up position and take a deep breath before moving on to the next exercise (an inhale and an exhale). Relax into a neutral position and then release the posture.

Advantages: Builds muscle in the arms, legs, and core. Increases the level of coordination.

## With weights, do single knee raises?

Beginning Position: In Mountain Pose, sit up straight and place both weights on your right knee. This is your starting position.

Movement: While resting your right hand over the two weights to keep them in position, gently raise your right knee straight up, and then slowly return your foot to the floor. Repeat this movement. Repeat this process ten times. Hold your leg high and take a deep breath as you complete the last repetition. Put your foot back down on the ground, and then swap sides. Next, put the two weights on your left knee where your kneecap would typically be.

Repetition: Perform this movement ten times on each side. On the very final repetition of each side, you should be sure to take a complete breath before beginning the next one. Release posture.

Advantages: It helps strengthen your quadriceps.

## Sit-stand up.

To begin, make sure you are sitting up straight in your chair.

Position your hands, so they are resting on the armrests of the chair you are sitting in. Then, while keeping your back straight and bending forward slightly, gaze ahead without turning your head. Now stand approximately six inches taller than you were in the chair, and then return to sitting.

Eight times is the recommended number of repetitions for this exercise. If getting out of the chair isn't difficult for you, you may try standing with your arms stretched completely straight out in front of you while you do so.

Benefits: Strengthens the gluteus muscles responsible for controlling sitting and standing positions. Increases overall sense of equilibrium.

Let's stop once again, and every one of us should take three deep breaths. First, take a deep and steady breath through your nose, and then slowly and steadily let out your breath through your mouth.

## Point and Flex with a Single-Leg

Begin by taking a lofty position in your chair with your back completely straight.

Movement: While taking a deep breath, stretch your right leg in front of you straight. While maintaining this stance for your other leg, start pointing your right foot and flexing it. This may be done at a gradual pace or a fast one. In any case, you are giving your foot and ankle excellent exercise. Next, put your hands in whichever position is most at ease for you, whether down by your sides or in your lap. To the best of your ability, emphasize both the point and the flex. After you have completed the task, put your foot back on the ground and swap sides.

The number of repetitions is fifteen times on each side. Repeat.

In addition to strengthening the foot and ankle, this exercise stretches the shin and calf muscles.

## Single-Leg Ankle Circles

Mountain Pose is the starting position. Sit as tall as you can in your chair.

Movement: While inhaling, raise your right leg and begin to twist your foot clockwise. Continue to hold this position for the duration of the movement. The circles should be articulated slowly. Make sure they are as oversized and dramatic as you can make them. After around ten revolutions, you should change the direction you're going in. Maintain as much straightness in your elevated leg as you can. Swap out the legs.

Ten sets on each side constitute one repetition.

The benefits include increased mobility as well as strengthened ankles.

## Each of the Legs Points and Bends

Sit in the "Mountain Pose" as the starting position.

Movement: While taking a deep breath, stretch both legs in front of you straight. While maintaining this stance with your legs, proceed to point and flex each of your feet. This may be done at a gradual pace or a fast one. In any case, you are giving your feet and ankles excellent exercise. Put your hands in whichever position is most at ease, whether down by your sides or in your lap. To the best of your ability, emphasize both the point and the flex. When you are completed, place both feet flat on the ground.

Repeat this process a total of fifteen times.

In addition to strengthening the feet and ankles, this exercise stretches the shin and calf muscles.

## Back Bend

Mountain Pose is the starting position. Come into it.

Move your hands, so they are resting on your legs with your palms facing down. Inhale slowly and steadily as you elevate your chest, gently arch your back, open your shoulders, and look upward toward the ceiling while you do so. While you are exhaling, bring your eyes down to the ground as you gently lower your head, round your back, and your shoulders. Now you should go back to neutral. Let's go back and try it again. When you inhale, ensure that you simultaneously lift your chest, arch your back, open your shoulders, and look up. Then, when you exhale, ensure you are doing the same thing. Some practice may be required, but the results will be well worth it.

Repeat this stance five times over your whole practice.

Advantages: It helps to warm up the lumbar and thoracic spine (upper and lower back). Encourages a healthy posture.

## Twist in the Chair

Position to begin: Sit up straight with your feet about hip-width apart.

Movement: Starting in an upright position, slowly rotate your upper body to the right and place your right hand on the top of the chair's back. Position your left hand such that it is on the outside of your right knee. Check that the front of both of your knees is facing the same direction. Lift your spine as you inhale, and then exhale as you gently twist to the right as you continue to twist. Get back to the neutral position. It takes considerable work to achieve this stance. Make sure that your lower body does not move at all!

The repetitions are as follows: Repeat five times on each side.

Benefits include massaging the internal organs and tightening the abdominal muscles.

Let's stop once again, and every one of us should take three deep breaths. First, take a deep and steady breath through your nose, and then slowly and steadily let out your breath through your mouth.

## Extend(ing) Their Arms Perform palm rotations while holding weights

Starting Position: Shoulders back and spine straight in Mountain Pose, with weights resting in hands on your lap. This is your starting position.

Movement: Extend both arms straight to the sides of your body with your palms facing upward. Each of your hands is now holding a weight. Maintain an extended stance with your arms and turn your palms down. Make sure that the only part of you moving is your palms, and then go from having your hands facing up to having them facing down.

Perform ten sets of repetitions.

The benefits include building strength in the arms and warming up the shoulders.

## Single-Leg Lifts with Weights

Beginning Position: While maintaining an elevated sitting position in Mountain Pose, place both weights on the upper part of your right leg, very near the knee.

Please perform the following movement by extending your right leg to the side and keeping it as straight as possible. Next, place your right hand on top of the two weights, and while maintaining this posture, gently raise one of your legs off the chair. When you lift anything, be sure your back is straight.

Lift your straight leg ten times to each side. This will be one repetition. At the tenth repetition on each side, hold the raised leg for one whole breath as you lower the other leg. Release.

Benefits: Strengthens muscles throughout the wide leg.

## Heel Raises

The starting position consists of sitting tall and pointing both feet forward.

To do this movement, ensure that your toes are

firmly placed on the floor, then proceed to elevate your heels. Maintain the lift in your heels while keeping your toes planted firmly on the ground. Exaggerate the heel lift with each repetition if you can do so comfortably.

Repeat this process a total of fifteen times.

Benefits: It stretches the muscles in your calves.

## Toe Raises

First, ensure that you sit straight and your feet point in front of you.

To do this movement, ensure that your heels are securely placed on the ground and elevate your toes. Maintain the lift on your toes while ensuring that your heels stay firmly on the floor. Exaggerate the lift each time, but only if you feel comfortable doing so.

Repeat this process a total of fifteen times.

The shins are stretched out, which is a benefit.

## Toe Squeeze

Sit in the "Mountain Pose" as the starting position.

Movement: Bring both legs forward and out to the sides while inhaling. Hold them in place as you pinch your toes together as firmly as you can, then let go of the pressure and spread your toes as far apart as you can. Crunch once more, making sure that everything is as compact as possible! After that, let it loose and spread. Imagine that you can stretch your toes so far apart that none of your toes are in contact with one another. In reality, this is only something to strive toward in the future. One or two of your toes will probably contact.

Repetition: Do this at least fifteen times in total. It's such a nice feeling!

The toes, feet, and ankles will all benefit from this stretch.

## Everything Dependent upon the Weights

Beginning Position: You have reached the last iteration of Mountain Pose for this chair yoga session lasting twenty minutes. Make it a memorable experience. Maintain an elevated sitting position with your knees hip distance apart, and your toes pointed forward. Hold your stomach in toward your spine. Keep weight in each hand and place them on your lower legs as support.

Lifting your arms and legs simultaneously when inhaling is the exercise's movement. You are in control of the weights. Make an effort to keep all your limbs and your back as straight as possible while maintaining comfort. Exhale, then bring your arms and legs back to the beginning position as gently as possible.

Repetition: Hold this stance a total of eight times. Hold the stance for the last repetition while taking in a complete breath. Release.

Benefits: Builds strength throughout the whole body.

## Position for Deep Relaxation

Position to Start: Lie on the seat, so the chair supports your back. Put your hands in a position of comfort on your lap, and then shut your eyes.

Movement: Take nice, easy breaths and relax every muscle in your body. Permit yourself to relax all the muscles in your face, shoulders, legs, and feet.

Repetitions: Maintain this comfortable posture for around five minutes while breathing in a natural and unforced manner.

Advantages: It makes it possible for your body to take in all of the positive effects of your yoga practice.

Let's take three nice, deep breaths right now. Take a deep and steady breath through your nose, and then slowly and steadily let out your breath through your mouth. You have just finished an exercise that will completely transform your life if you do it at least three times a week. Congratulations! Great work.

# Increasing the time

I am delighted you are prepared to go on to the intermediate routine that lasts thirty minutes. It is a significant obligation to fulfill. It is going to take a lot of effort and self-control. Is there going to be a problem? First, let's get ourselves warmed up.

Position yourself in the beginning stage of the mountain pose by sitting up straight and tall on your chair, keeping your knees hip-width apart, and pointing your toes in a forward direction. Put your hands on your thighs while you do this. To improve your posture, roll your shoulders up and down your back, and bring your navel into your spine.

## The breath

Come to sit in Mountain Pose, which is the starting position.

Movement: Inhale slowly and steadily through your nose, and expel slowly and steadily through your mouth. This is one complete breath. Do not try to force your breath. Instead, it would help if you worked toward making the exhale duration equal to that of the inhale. For example, you may begin by counting to two on the inhale and then counting to two on the exhale to get you started. If you can make the pause between each inhale and exhale longer, for example, a count of three to four, then you should try to do so.

Repeatedly take four full breaths before continuing. Don't forget to go slow and steady.

The benefits of using this breathing style include reducing anxiety and calming the nervous system. In addition, it gets your muscles ready for action.

## Side Neck Bend

Mountain Pose is the starting position. Come into it.

Movement: Take a deep breath in and sit up straight. As you let your breath out, bring the right ear down to the right shoulder. Check to see that your shoulders are loose and relaxed. Next, take a deep breath to restore equilibrium to your brain. Now, take a deep breath to help you sit up straight, and then let out your breath as you bring your left ear to your left shoulder. Again, take a deep breath to restore equilibrium to your brain. This is one of the sets.

Perform the set three times in a row as your repetitions.

The sides of the neck are stretched out, which is a benefit.

## Neck Turns

To return to the starting position, assume the mountain pose.

Movement: While inhaling, gradually rotate to the right with your head. As you let your breath out, come back to the center of your body very gently. While you are breathing in, gently move your head to the left. Return to the center while exhaling in a leisurely and even manner.

Perform the set three times in a row as your repetitions.

Benefits: Helps to restore mobility in the upper back and reduces stress in the neck and shoulders.

## Shoulder Shrugs

Mountain Pose is the starting position. Resume this pose.

Inhale as you pull both of your shoulders up to your ears and exhale as you return them to their neutral position at the beginning of the movement. Then, increase the amount of the lift.

Repeat this process a total of five times.

Advantages: Reduces the amount of strain on the neck and shoulders muscles.

Rings on the Wrists

Mountain Pose is the starting position. Sit up as tall as you can. Place your belly button in line with your spine and draw the crown of your head up toward the ceiling as you sit.

Movement: Keep your elbows tight to your sides and reach your hands out in front of you while doing this action. Roll your hands around at the wrists while extending all of your fingers. Move your fingers around while simultaneously rolling your wrists.

Repetitions: Roll your wrists in one way, then switch and roll ten times in the other direction.

Advantages: Warms up the hands, including the wrists and fingers. Additionally reduces inflammation in the joints of the hand.

# Raise your arms above using both of them.

Take the position known as "Mountain Pose" to begin.

Movement: Raise both arms over your head while maintaining a calm and steady inhalation. Exhale slowly and steadily as you bring your arms back to the beginning position. During movement, make sure your shoulders remain relaxed. If you find raising your arms above difficult, you should lift them to a more comfortable level.

Repetition: You will need to do this five times.

Advantages: Promotes shoulder joint flexibility and builds arms' strength.

## Knee Swings

Position yourself in Mountain Pose, with your shoulders back, and your tummy tucked up, and sit up tall.

Move your hands such that they are clasped beneath your right knee. Maintain an upright posture with a spine that is straight. While maintaining this position, kick your leg to the side in a back and forth motion. This is one of the few poses that we can do rather rapidly. If you cannot reach under your knee, you should lean back in the chair and kick out your right leg while swinging it back and forth at a reasonable pace. Again, if you cannot reach under your knee, you should continue with the next step.

The recommended number of repetitions for each leg is twenty.

Gains in mobility and range of motion in the knees are among the benefits.

## Complete a set of ankle circles with both legs

Mountain Pose is the starting position. Come into it.

Movement: While inhaling, elevate your spine and stretch both legs as far as you comfortably can. To attain this stance, ensure you are seated back in your chair. While trying to keep your legs completely straight, begin to spin your feet and ankles in a clockwise direction. Your feet and ankles are the only portions of your body that move when you sleep.

Perform ten revolutions in each direction to

complete one repetition.

Benefits: Increases range of motion in the feet and ankles

We have now reached the end of our warm-up! Let's begin our practice.

## Rolls with the Hands on the Shoulders

Mountain Pose is the starting position, so come into that.

Movement: With your hands resting on top of your shoulders, move your shoulders in huge circles while guiding them with your elbows. Maintain a relaxed breathing pattern as you move. Alter the direction in which your circles are going.

Repeat steps one through eight times in each direction.

The benefits include relaxing the stiffness in your neck and warming up your upper back.

## Shoulder Twists and Rolls

Mountain Pose is the starting position. Sit up as tall as you can.

Inhale as you raise your shoulders and back, and exhale as you return them to the beginning position. Movement: Inhale as you lift your shoulders up and back. Create as much of a seamless circle as possible with the movement by making it as fluid as possible. After you have completed five calm and steady circles, switch directions. As you inhale, push your shoulders toward your body as you lift them, and as you exhale, return your shoulders to their beginning position behind your neck. This course of action is inherently uncomfortable. You don't need to worry about it since you're already doing it right!

The exercise should be performed eight times in each direction. The repetitions

Advantages: Increases flexibility and range of motion while opening the shoulder joints.

## Bending Forward While Maintaining a Straight Back

Position yourself in the starting position by sitting up straight in your chair and placing your hands on top of your thighs.

Movement: Bring your chin to your chest as you inhale and bend forward from the hips. Always remember to have a straight spine. It would help if you only went as far as possible while keeping a straight back. The hips are where the bend begins. As you exhale, rise back to a standing position by placing your hands on your knees and utilizing them to propel you upward. Maintain your gaze on the path directly before you during the movement. Do not stare at your feet. This movement may not be significant, depending on how flexible your spine is. That is not in the least bit problematic. Keep in mind that the movement is quite sluggish!

Repeat this process a total of eight times. Hold the bent posture for the eighth repetition while taking one complete breath that consists of a slow, steady intake and a slow, steady exhale. This is one whole breath. Get back to being neutral.

Advantages: Increases flexibility in the back while simultaneously strengthening the muscles in the lower back

## Arm Raises interspersed with Weighted Exercises

Come into Mountain Pose while holding the two-pound weights in each hand and letting them rest on your thighs. This is your starting position.

Only do this action if it does not cause discomfort by lifting your right arm over your head while inhaling. If it isn't, you should elevate your arm as high as it is comfortable to go. Make an effort to maintain the straight position of your extended arm while keeping your shoulder relaxed. As you bring your arm closer to your body, exhale. Turn the other cheek.

Repetition: You will need to do this six times on each side. On the last repetition on each side, hold the posture and be sure to take two deep breaths. Relax into the posture, then go back to the starting position. Throughout the workout, you are holding the weights in both hands.

Advantages include arm strengthening as well as lubrication of the shoulder joint.

## Rotation of the trunk while holding weights in extended arms

Mountain Pose is the starting position; hold weights in both hands and assume this position.

Movement: While holding a weight in each hand, begin by extending your arms to the sides of your body as you inhale. Exhale. While you are inhaling, gently rotate to your right. Your head moves in the same direction as your right arm when stretched. Exhale and come back to the center. Keep your arms at your sides. If you are using a mirror, you should ensure that your shoulders are relaxed and that your arms are at shoulder level as you stretch them. Take a deep breath in and rotate to your left. The left arm is responsible for transporting your head. Bring your arms down until resting on your legs, and then return to the neutral position.

The repetitions are as follows: Perform each set eight times. Maintain the stance for the last repetition on each side, taking two full breaths as you do so. Relax into the posture, then go back to the starting position.

Advantages: Slims the waistline and builds strength in the arms.

Let's stop for a moment and take three deep breaths together. First, take a deep and steady breath through your nose, and then slowly and steadily let out your breath through your mouth.

## Exercise for the Side of the Body Using Weights

Assume a good and lofty Mountain Pose sitting position as a starting position. Next, place the weights in each of your hands on your thighs.

Inhale as you pull both arms up and maintain this position while holding weights in both hands. Movement: Exhale. As you take your next breath, tilt your body to the right. As you bring your arms back to the neutral position, exhale as you do so. At the same time, you are inhaling slowly and steadily, lean to your left side while keeping your arms up over your head. As you bring both arms back up to the overhead position, exhale.

Perform a total of eight sets of repetitions. The arms remain up throughout. Hold the posture for the last repetition on each side, and take two deep breaths. Relax into the posture, then go back to the starting position.

Benefits: Tones waistline.

## Bicep Curls with Weights, Performing Alternating Arms

Come to a sitting position in Mountain Pose with the weights in your hands. This is your starting position.

Movement: Bring your arms down to your sides and rest them there. Maintain a position in which your elbows are firmly affixed to the sides of your body. Your right arm should be bent up gently as you inhale, and you should exhale as it is lowered back to the starting position. Take a deep breath as you raise your left arm, and then let out as you lower it back to the starting position. Throughout the action, your elbows will remain firmly planted at your sides.

The repetitions are as follows: repeat each side eight times. Then, after taking a hiatus, continue the exercise for eight repetitions on each side.

Biceps muscle may be built up with regular use of this product.

# Raise your arms and legs individually using weights

Mountain Pose is the starting position. Bring some weights onto your lap and come into Mountain Pose.

Movement: Take a deep breath as you raise your right leg and right arm (the weight should be in your hand). Your arm and your leg have to be as straight as you possibly can get them to be. As you bring them down, exhale as you do so.

Repetition: You will need to do this six times on each side. On the last repetition of each side, hold the posture in the up position and take two deep breaths before moving on to the next side. Relax into a neutral position and then release the posture.

Advantages: Builds muscle in the arms, legs, and core. Increases the level of coordination.

# With weights, do single knee raises?

Beginning Position: In Mountain Pose, sit up straight and place both weights on your right knee.

This is your starting position.

Movement: While resting your right hand over the two weights to keep them in position, gently raise your right knee straight up, and then slowly return your foot to the floor. Repeat this movement. Repeat this process ten times. Hold your knee-high, and take two deep breaths before moving on to the last repetition. Put your foot back down on the ground, and then swap sides. Next, put the two weights on your left knee where your kneecap would typically be.

Repetition: Perform this movement ten times on each side. During the last repetition of each side, be sure to keep your knee in the up position and take two deep breaths. Release posture.

Advantages: It helps strengthen your quadriceps.

## Sit-stand up.

To begin, make sure you are sitting up straight in your chair.

Position your hands, so they are resting on the armrests of the chair you are sitting in. Then, while keeping your back straight and bending forward slightly, gaze ahead without turning your head. Now stand approximately six inches taller than you were in the chair, and then return to sitting.

Eight times is the recommended number of

repetitions for this exercise. If getting out of the chair isn't difficult for you, you may try standing with your arms stretched completely straight out in front of you while you do so.

Benefits: Strengthens the gluteus muscles responsible for controlling sitting and standing positions. Increases overall sense of equilibrium.

Let's stop once again, and every one of us should take three deep breaths. First, take a deep and steady breath through your nose, and then slowly and steadily let out your breath through your mouth.

## Point and Flex with a Single-Leg

Begin by taking a lofty position in your chair with your back completely straight.

Movement: While taking a deep breath, stretch your right leg in front of you straight. While maintaining this stance for your other leg, start pointing your right foot and flexing it. This may be done at a gradual pace or a fast one. In any case, you are giving your foot and ankle excellent exercise. Next, put your hands in whichever position is most at ease for you, whether down by your sides or in your lap. To the best of your ability, emphasize both the point and the flex. After you have completed the task, put your foot back on the ground and swap sides.

The number of repetitions is fifteen times on each side. Repeat.

In addition to strengthening the foot and ankle, this exercise stretches the shin and calf muscles.

Single-Leg Ankle Circles

Mountain Pose is the starting position. Sit as tall as you can in your chair.

Movement: While inhaling, raise your right leg and begin to twist your foot clockwise. Continue to hold this position for the duration of the movement. The circles should be articulated slowly. Make sure they are as oversized and dramatic as you can make them. After around ten revolutions, you should change the direction you're going in. Maintain as much straightness in your elevated leg as you can. Swap out the legs.

Ten sets on each side constitute one repetition.

The benefits include increased mobility as well as strengthened ankles.

## Each of the Legs Points and Bends

Sit in the "Mountain Pose" as the starting position.

Movement: While taking a deep breath, stretch both legs in front of you straight. While maintaining this stance with your legs, proceed to point and flex each of your feet. This may be done at a gradual pace or a fast one. In any case, you are giving your feet and ankles excellent exercise. Put your hands in whichever position is most at ease, whether down by your sides or in your lap. To the best of your ability, emphasize both the point and the flex. When you are completed, place both feet flat on the ground.

Repeat this process a total of fifteen times.

In addition to strengthening the feet and ankles, this exercise stretches the shin and calf muscles.

## Back Bend

Mountain Pose is the starting position. Come into it.

Move your hands, so they are resting on your legs with your palms facing down. Inhale slowly and steadily as you elevate your chest, gently arch your back, open your shoulders, and look upward toward the ceiling while you do so. While you are exhaling, bring your eyes down to the ground as you gently lower your head, round your back, and your shoulders. Now you should go back to neutral. Let's go back and try it again. When you inhale, ensure that you simultaneously lift your chest, arch your back, open your shoulders, and look up. Then, when you exhale, ensure you are doing the same thing. Some practice may be required, but the results will be well worth it.

Repeat this stance five times over your whole practice.

Advantages: It helps to warm up the lumbar and thoracic spine (upper and lower back). Encourages a healthy posture.

## Twist in the Chair

Position to begin: Sit up straight with your feet about hip-width apart.

Movement: Starting in an upright position, slowly rotate your upper body to the right and place your right hand on the top of the chair's back. Position your left hand such that it is on the outside of your right knee. Check that the front of both of your knees is facing the same direction. Lift your spine as you inhale, and then exhale as you gently twist to the right as you continue to twist. Get back to the neutral position. It takes considerable work to achieve this stance. Make sure that your lower body does not move at all!

The repetitions are as follows: Repeat five times on each side.

Benefits include massaging the internal organs and tightening the abdominal muscles.

## Extend(ing) Their Arms Perform palm rotations while holding weights

Starting Position: Shoulders back and spine straight in Mountain Pose, with weights resting in hands on your lap. This is your starting position.

Movement: Extend both arms straight to the sides of your body with your palms facing upward. Each of your hands is now holding a weight. Maintain an extended stance with your arms and turn your palms down. Make sure that the only part of you moving is your palms, and then go from having your hands facing up to having them facing down.

Perform ten sets of repetitions.

The benefits include building strength in the arms and warming up the shoulders.

## Single-Leg Lifts with Weights

Beginning Position: While maintaining an elevated sitting position in Mountain Pose, place both weights on the upper part of your right leg, very near your knee.

Perform the following movement by extending your right leg to the side and keeping it as straight as possible. Next, place your right hand on top of the two weights, and while maintaining this posture, gently raise one of your legs off the chair. When you lift anything, be sure your back is straight.

Lifting your straight leg eight times on each side is the prescribed number of repetitions. Hold the raised leg for two breaths at the eighth repetition on each side while doing the exercise. Release.

Benefits: Strengthens muscles throughout the wide leg.

## Heel Raises

The starting position consists of sitting tall and pointing both feet forward.

To do this movement, ensure that your toes are firmly placed on the floor, then proceed to elevate your heels. Maintain the lift in your heels while keeping your toes planted firmly on the ground. Exaggerate the heel lift with each repetition if you can do so comfortably.

Repeat this process a total of fifteen times.

Benefits: It stretches the muscles in your calves.

## Toe Raises

First, ensure that you sit straight and your feet point in front of you.

To do this movement, ensure that your heels are securely placed on the ground and elevate your toes. Then, maintain the lift on your toes while ensuring that your heels stay planted firmly on the floor. Exaggerate the lift each time, but only if you feel comfortable doing so.

Repeat this process a total of fifteen times.

The shins are stretched out, which is a benefit.

## Toe Squeeze

Sit in the "Mountain Pose" as the starting position.

Movement: Bring both legs forward and out to the sides while inhaling. Hold them in place as you pinch your toes together as firmly as you can, then let go of the pressure and spread your toes as far apart as you can. Crunch once more, making sure that everything is as compact as possible! After that, let it loose and spread. Imagine that you can stretch your toes so far apart that none of your toes are in contact with one another. In reality, this is only something to strive toward in the future. One or two of your toes will probably contact.

Repetition: Do this at least fifteen times in total. It's

such a nice feeling!

The toes, feet, and ankles will all benefit from this stretch.

## Everything Dependent upon the Weights

Beginning Position: You have reached the end of your mountain pose sequence for your chair yoga practice that lasted thirty minutes. Make it a memorable experience. Maintain an elevated sitting position with your knees hip distance apart, and your toes pointed forward. Hold your stomach in toward your spine. Keep weight in each hand and place them on your lower legs as support.

Lifting your arms and legs simultaneously when inhaling is the exercise's movement. You are in control of the weights. Make an effort to keep all your limbs and your back as straight as possible while maintaining comfort. Exhale, then bring your arms and legs back to the beginning position as gently as possible.

Repetition: Hold this stance a total of eight times. Hold the posture for the last repetition while taking in two full breaths. Release.

Benefits: Builds strength throughout the whole body.

## Position for Deep Relaxation

Position to Start: Lie on the seat, so the chair supports your back. Put your hands in a position of comfort on your lap, and then shut your eyes.

Movement: Take nice, easy breaths and relax every muscle in your body. Permit yourself to relax all the muscles in your face, shoulders, legs, and feet.

Repetitions: Maintain this comfortable posture for around five minutes while breathing in a natural and unforced manner.

Advantages: It makes it possible for your body to take in all of the positive effects of your yoga practice.

Take three deep breaths in and out. First, take a deep and steady breath through your nose, and then slowly and steadily let out your breath through your mouth.

This is a very significant accomplishment. You just finished a strenuous chair yoga program that lasted for thirty minutes. The most challenging aspect is committing to it at least three times weekly. This should not become a routine! A healthy and wholesome routine.

# Positions While Standing

## 1. Forward Fold

Method: Place yourself about one foot away from the chair and face it, so its back is facing you. Put your hands on the chair's back to steady yourself.

Keep your knees over your ankles and your hips over your knees as you go forward from your hips into a bending position.

Hold.

Try rotating the chair around, so the seat is facing you if you find this position comfortable.

Put your hands on the chair seat and lean forward

from the hips until you can reach the seat.

Duration: Maintain this position for five calm breaths.

Caution: Avoid making this motion if it causes you to experience strain or discomfort.

Check that your back and neck are both in a straight position.

Always make sure you move gently and carefully, bending from your hips and using your core muscles.

Advantages: Increases the range of motion in the hip joints.

Activates and stretches the muscles in the posterior region of the thighs.

# 2. Raised Knee Balance

Stand with the side of the chair facing you while doing the Raised Knee Balance Method.

Make sure that your whole foot is resting on the chair's seat after you place the foot closest to the chair on top of the seat.

Maintain your equilibrium by grabbing hold of the chair's back.

If your equilibrium is sound, try raising your hand

an inch or two off the back of the chair and seeing how it feels.

Duration: Maintain this position for five calm breaths.

Caution: Avoid making this motion if it causes you to experience strain or discomfort.

If the chair is too high for you, you may get better balance by turning it around and resting your foot on a stool or block. Keep in mind that you should always move gently and deliberately.

Advantages: Increases the range of motion in the hip and knee joints. Strengthens the muscles in the leg that is in the standing position. Enhances one's equilibrium.

# 3. Hip Half-Circle

Stand with your left hip near the back of the chair and your left hand holding onto the chair. This is the Hip Half-Circle Method.

Move your right foot forward and toward the chair while maintaining the straight position of your right leg.

Forward.

To the side of the road.

Back.

To the side of the road.

Forward.

In the direction of the chair and forward.

Duration: You will need to complete this cycle five times.

Perform the whole sequence with the leg that is opposite your dominant leg.

Caution: Avoid making this motion if it causes you to experience strain or discomfort. Keep in mind that you should always move gently and deliberately.

Advantages: Increases the range of motion in the hip joints.

Increases the muscular endurance of the standing leg via improved strength.

Enhances one's equilibrium.

# 4. On Your Tiptoes

Method: Turn your back to the front of the chair.

Put your hands on the chair's back to steady yourself.

Rise onto your tiptoes.

Check to see whether you can lift and drop your heels in the most measured and discreet manner possible.

Duration:

Repeat between 5 and ten times.

Precautions:

Do not continue if you are experiencing strain or discomfort from this activity.

When your heels do hit the floor, there should be no impact felt by your feet.

Advantages:

Increases the range of motion in the joints of the ankles.

Increases the foot's range of motion.

Strengthens the muscles in the calf and improves overall performance.

Enhances one's equilibrium.

5. A Stretch for the Calf

Step one of the method is to roll up a tiny towel and lay it on the floor behind the chair after unrolling it.

You should put your hands on the back of the chair while you are standing behind it.

Put one foot in front of the other.

You should maintain the heel of this foot on the floor as you rest the ball of this foot on the towel.

Make sure that your hips are pulled back and that they are directly over the heel of the leg that you are extending.

Duration:

Maintain this position for five calm breaths.

Perform the same action with the opposite foot.

Caution:

Avoid making this motion if it causes you to experience strain or discomfort.

Maintain a flat heel on the floor with the calf you are extending.

Calves are lengthened as a result of this benefit.

Increases the range of motion in the ankle joint.

Enhances one's equilibrium.

6. Rising from a seated position

The method is to rise from a sitting position while maintaining as much composure and slowness as possible.

Take a seat once again.

If you need to, you may either keep your hands on the seat or stretch your arms in front of you.

Duration:

Perform at least five times in total.

Caution:

Avoid making this motion if it causes you to experience strain or discomfort.

You may set a chair in front of you and use it to assist you in getting to your feet if you feel like you have an inferior balance.

Advantages: This exercise aims to develop the ability to deliberately transition from a seated to a standing position and back.

# 7. From the Ground Up to Standing

Method: Position yourself next to the chair.

Make your way down onto the floor and into a sitting posture by using the chair.

Make your way back to a standing posture by using the chair.

If you face the seat toward yourself, the chair will be far less likely to tip over.

Duration: Perform at least five times in total.

Caution: Avoid making this motion if it causes you to experience strain or discomfort.

Put down a yoga mat on the floor where you will be sitting if you regularly get sore knees.

Advantages: This is a helpful workout for increasing the strength necessary to get up off the floor, and this exercise focuses on your core. The development of this ability is essential given that there are circumstances in which we may find ourselves unbalanced and need assistance getting back up off the ground.

If you can only consistently commit to doing one exercise from this complete regimen, make it this one. It will provide you with the most bang for your buck.

## 8. Tree

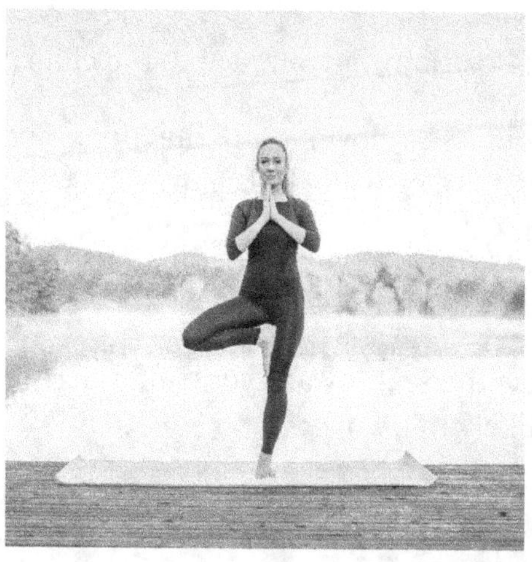

The method calls for you to place your left hand on

the back of the chair while standing behind it. Then, raise the knee on your right side while keeping your right hand on your hip.

Put the sole of your right foot on your left leg below your knee, or rest the toes of your right foot on the ground while resting your right heel on your left thigh. Alternatively, put the sole of your right foot on your left leg above your knee.

If you are feeling stable, try raising one hand off the chair by an inch or bringing both hands together in front of your chest. If none of these seems suitable, try shifting your weight slightly.

Duration: maintain balance for roughly five deep breaths in a calm state.

Perform the same movement with the opposite leg.

Caution: Avoid making this motion if it causes you to experience strain or discomfort.

When your right sole is up against your left leg, check to see that it is positioned such that it is resting below the knee. As a result, there shouldn't be any pressure from the side pressing on your knee when standing.

Advantages: Increases the range of motion in the hip joints.

Enhances one's equilibrium.

Boosts one's awareness of their own body.

Boosts the muscular endurance of the leg that is standing.

## 9. Warrior I

The method calls for you to place your feet hip-width apart and stand behind the chair.

Bring your right foot back as far as possible while maintaining complete contact with the ground with both feet. Your second toe should be pointing out to the side ever-so-slightly.

You should move your hips closer to the chair while bending your front knee.

You should loosen up your shoulders.

Check that both of your hips are pointed in the direction of the chair.

Both of your feet need to be planted entirely on the ground. If you cannot maintain your rear foot firmly planted on the ground, you should shift it forward a few inches.

Maintain a straight line from your shoulders to your hips.

If you are not experiencing discomfort, you may want to try resting your hands on your hips or raising one or both of your arms over your head.

Hold for a duration of roughly five breaths while remaining calm.

On the other side, repeat the process.

Caution: Avoid making this motion if it causes you to experience strain or discomfort.

Be confident that your front knee does not extend farther than your front ankle; instead, your front knee should be positioned immediately above your front ankle.

Advantages: Increases the range of motion in the hip and knee joints.

Enhances one's equilibrium.

Boosts one's awareness of their own body.

Leg strength is improved with this exercise.

# You can do this anywhere!

When you finally get into the swing of things with your exercise program, I think you'll conclude that next to spending time with family and friends, maintaining a regular exercise regimen is the essential thing you can do for yourself. In addition, maintaining an exercise routine helps you develop a more optimistic attitude on life and lessens feelings of worry and discomfort.

You will soon conclude that you can do most of these exercises in almost any place, which is the next step in the progression of this new aspect of your life. You don't need additional, and you need special equipment to

I was hoping you could permit me to assist you in working through this situation. When you are seated on a chair, whether it be at a friend's house, in the waiting room of a doctor's office, on an aircraft, on a bus, or as a passenger in a vehicle, you have the opportunity to move your body in ways that are helpful to your health. Because it is obvious that you do not want to draw any unwelcome attention to yourself, I will now provide a list of positions that you can do in understated ways that will contribute to the fitness level you have worked so diligently to obtain.

Mountain Posture was the first pose you learned on this page, and it is also, in many respects, the most significant one of all of the poses described here. Even if you are sitting on a sofa or a chair with a cushion, you can still sit up tall and straight by drawing your belly button in toward your spine, rising and opening your shoulders, keeping your knees and feet pointing straight forward, and maintaining a smooth and steady flow of breath. Furthermore, you can maintain this posture and way of breathing even if you are seated for a significant amount of time; all you have to do is keep going back to it.

Moving on from the Mountain Pose, let's work on releasing any stress or tension that may be held in our necks. This may be accomplished by using controlled rotations of the neck and side bending of the neck. This is the action from our warm-up routine that goes from the ear to the shoulder.

Shoulder rolls are a great way to loosen up tight

shoulders, so let's move down the list of postures from the primary series and try them.

The forward bend with a straight back is the next position, which always feels lovely in my body. Repeat this movement a few times while maintaining a calm and steady breath to feel a slight stretch in your spine.

Now let's talk about the bottom part of your body. Perform some Single-Leg lifts anywhere there is space in front of you—perhaps not in a moving vehicle or on an airplane, but most certainly elsewhere. Your circulation in your lower extremities will improve as a result of this. Knee lifts are another simple posture that can be performed in a seated position anywhere. The muscles that surround the knee joint are improved in strength as a result.

The postures for the feet come last, but they are certainly not the least important. We can execute each of these inconspicuously.

You should try a Single-Leg point and flex and a Single-Leg ankle circle. You may still carry out the exercises even if you cannot extend your leg straight before you; raise your foot a few inches off the ground and continue.

Last but not least, there are heel lifts, and toe raises, which are excellent for the health of your feet and can be readily performed anywhere you take a seat.

What happens if you are alone in your house, watching television or just unwinding by reading a book or magazine?

Experiment with knee swings, toe squeezes, wrist circles, ankle circles on both legs, pointing and flexing both legs, alternating arm lifts, and wrist circles. You are free to try any or all of the different stances. Go in order. Try doing things in reverse. Do three different positions. Just make sure that you are breathing deliberately. Take three deep breaths, maintaining a steady and calm pace. Do ten postures. Just perform toe squeezes.

Do you understand what I'm trying to say? Make an effort to move as much of your body as possible, regardless of where you are or what you are doing. Utilizing the information provided in this book, you should try to lengthen, stretch, and expand your muscles and joints. Thanks to the skills and knowledge you've gained, you have the resources necessary to accomplish and keep a healthy mind and body.

## Gather your friends

Have you been a dedicated practitioner of chair yoga for the last several months, to the point that you can't stop raving about it to anybody who will listen? I'm going to think that you are, and I'm also going to guess that some of the praise you've been receiving could have something to do with it. When we don't get enough physical activity, it shows in our faces, our bodies, how we move, and how we interact with others. It makes us feel more at ease and reduces the tension we experience. It is beneficial for this purpose when combined with the frequent practice of conscious breathing.

You have probably picked up on the fact that I use the term "habit" somewhat often. This is not a coincidental occurrence. Behavior that one engages in repeatedly without giving it any conscious thought becomes a habit. You can't help but comply with the demand placed upon you. A practice is not a habit if it is only done on occasion. A habit may be either beneficial or detrimental to one's life. Smoking is most likely the first example of a poor habit that most of us consider. Reading, being active, and volunteering are just a few examples of highly beneficial habits. I do not doubt that you may consider many such examples.

Maintaining the habit over time is essential to its success. A habit is formed by doing chair yoga at a frequency of at least three times per week. In addition, you may do a few other yoga positions at any point throughout the day, regardless of where you are seated. The key to success is consistency.

What exactly does this have to do with dividing things between your pals? If you have worked exercise into your routine and are aware of its advantages, it is only natural that you want to tell your friends about your experiences. When I say "share," I don't simply mean telling someone about your experience and urging them to give it a go, although that is part of what I mean. Instead, I propose getting a few people together to do the task at someone's house, whether yours or someone else's. So how do you do it? Here are some options.

Find an area large enough to hold a few seats all at once. I think it would be best to start this group journey with only one or two buddies, and then, if it goes well, you may add more people. Arrange the seats such that they create a horseshoe shape. This arrangement enables people to make eye contact with one another. When everyone is seated, check to see that they can stretch their arms and legs in all directions without colliding.

In a perfect world, each participant would have a copy of Chair Yoga for Seniors. If this does not occur, the instructions will be read by whomever currently has the book. Because you have been doing this for some time, you have likely committed the instructions to memory at this point. Refrain from doing this, though, since the people you have invited over will need to know all of the minute nuances to perform the postures correctly, and they will need your help.

Agree on the kind of music that will be played. There is a good chance that you and your pals like listening to music of the same style. Put your imagination to work. If somebody in your group uses Apple Music or Spotify, they might put up a lively playlist that you could listen to throughout your group sessions.

This ought to be an enjoyable activity. Establish some ground rules, but try not to be too harsh on one another. Don't stress about the appropriate moment. Spend as much time as is necessary for each person to comprehend the proper way to carry out each position. Because you, the reader, are responsible for bringing this group together, you must remind everyone to stay within their own range of mobility and avoid doing any activity that causes discomfort.

Everyone takes a sip of water, and then we'll start the warm-up exercises.

## feeling a lot better?

Since you've started doing chair yoga daily, I'm sure your loved ones have picked up on some of the changes that have taken place in you. You are breathing better, standing taller, moving with greater self-assurance, having a more positive attitude on life, and standing taller as a result. I hope that this has whetted your appetite for additional information. And what else? I will explain it to you. A vast array of options is accessible to us in the form of improvements and alterations to our way of life that may make our lives better, healthier, and more satisfying. Stay with me through the rest of this chapter if you are prepared to let more excellent health, happiness, satisfaction, purpose, and peace into your life, yourself, and the life you lead. Finally, I want to share some of the highlights of my trip with you in the hopes that they will encourage you to broaden your horizons.

If you are willing to investigate, I must ask you to bear with me while making a few assumptions about you. If you are ready to investigate, I will ask you to suffer with me. I guess that when you went out and got this book, one of your goals was to find something that would help you feel better. You probably began with the programs geared for beginners, and as your skills and self-assurance improved, you progressed to the programs described as intermediate in the book. You probably already include a chair yoga regimen into your everyday life at this point. In addition to preparing your home environment to go through a twenty- or thirty-minute program three or more times each week, you may move your neck, shoulders, legs, and feet in any sitting position. You feel terrific. You've come a long way in a short amount of time. You experience less tension and stress, and you are also better able to handle your aches and pains. Am I describing you? Or a different iteration of you? If you can identify with any of the specifics I have just outlined, you are prepared to open up your mind, heart, and body to live a genuinely holistic and healthy life.

I will discuss four successful activities with you via

extensive research and will significantly contribute to your life's enhancement in various ways. After that, I'll lead you through a thirty-minute advanced chair yoga and weight training program if you feel you're up for the challenge.

The following are the four areas that we shall look into:

• The benefits that come with maintaining a healthy diet.

• Some of the advantages of practicing meditation

• The advantages that come with volunteering.

• The importance of having strong social ties and communities.

## Healthy diet

Let's begin with maintaining a healthy diet, shall we? A dizzying array of advice on how to cut calories and lose weight can be found all over the media. It is often difficult to differentiate between content and advertisements on television. You may have meal plans sent to your home, extra protein drinks, supplements, and directions for when to eat, fast, and other things. It makes one feel queasy! There was never a food shortage in the typical Italian-American home where I spent my childhood. We were both encouraging one another to eat! The act of eating was a social occasion. So much attention is paid to food. It took me many decades to become less preoccupied with eating. I am still putting effort into it. I can keep my weight at a healthy level. However, I am having a hard time with it. I put a lot of different approaches to losing weight to the test throughout the years whenever I saw that the number on the scale was getting higher. Keeping a healthy diet has proven to be my most effective strategy.

What does it mean to have a healthy diet? The Mediterranean diet is one of the only diets endorsed by almost every health professional. It is more accurate to call this a lifestyle than a diet. It is associated with a risk reduction for cardiovascular disease of twenty-five percent. People with type 2 diabetes are another group that often receives this recommendation.

What foods make up a typical portion of a Mediterranean diet? It is a plant-based diet, with protein consumed as a "side." This involves eating a lot of fruits and vegetables, limiting your intake of skinless poultry and fish, and eating legumes, nuts, and healthy fats like olive oil and avocados in moderate quantities. Sweets and alcohol are permitted, but only in restricted quantities. Do you have any questions about bread and pasta? I am well aware of this fact. Whole grains! This is a must. It is vital to ensure that the bread you consume is prepared with whole grains. Examine the product package. Whole wheat is not the same thing as flour made from wheat. Be sure that the grain is being described using the term "whole" at all times. This also applies to pasta dishes. Pasta made from whole wheat is tasty and relatively easy to get in supermarkets and on menus.

If you want to lose some weight, you should cut down on foods that include whole grains, such as bread and pasta, and nuts. This is because all of them have a high-calorie count.

Oldwayspt.org is a fantastic online resource that provides information on the Mediterranean diet and how to follow it. Oldways developed the Mediterranean Diet Pyramid in 1993 in collaboration with the Harvard School of Public Health and the World Health Organization (WHO) as a more nutritious alternative to the original food pyramid developed by the USDA. It has all the knowledge that you need to understand how to pursue this as a lifestyle and why you should do so.

# Meditation

If you have never tried it before, you will probably write off meditation as some kind of new-age activity that isn't for you. I would want to dispel any preconceptions that you may have about meditating and then expose you to something that will benefit your capacity to deal with stressful situations and feel serene, all while decreasing your blood pressure and pulse rate! I'm aware that it seems too remarkable to be true. However, this is a fact.

In its most basic form, the core idea behind meditation is to give your brain a break from the myriad of ideas that constantly swirl through your head while you're awake. It takes just five minutes a day to practice, yet even that little amount of time may have positive results because of how easy it is to accomplish. Meditation is most beneficial when practiced consistently, much like an exercise routine. By devoting between five and ten minutes of each day to a meditation practice, you will be able to lessen the tension caused by the various obstacles we encounter as we get older and redirect that stress away from despair and sleeplessness.

How do you do it? Find a relaxing area to sit where your back will be supported, and you can feel completely at ease before continuing. Remove the cross you've made with your legs and arms, then put your hands in your lap. You should use a timer in the beginning stages of developing a regular meditation practice. You should use a kitchen timer, a stopwatch, or any other device that allows you to set the timer for at least five minutes.

Relax both your physical self and your mental self. You should begin with your eyes open, but your concentration should be gentle. First, give yourself a few good, deep breaths, and then slowly shut your eyes. Take regular, deep breaths. Pay attention to the sensations that are occurring in your body. You should begin at your head and work your way down your body. Take a few calm breaths. Observe how, as you breathe in, your stomach stretches out, and as you breathe out, your shoulders relax. Don't be concerned if random ideas start popping into your head. Bring your focus back slowly to the breath you are taking in and out. When you inhale, the air enters your body, and when you exhale, the air exits your body. You may think of this as the air entering and leaving your body. Another option is to think of yourself saying, "I am breathing in" and "I am breathing out." This will help you return to a calm state and center you in your meditation. You should gently open your eyes and take in the surroundings when the allotted time has passed.

Many individuals find that doing so simultaneously each day makes it much simpler to maintain a meditation practice. If this isn't something that would work for you, do it whenever you have five to ten minutes of peace to spare.

Suppose you are interested in trying out a variety of meditation techniques. In that case, I strongly suggest you download the Headspace app, which is accessible for free on both Apple and Android devices, or search for guided meditations on YouTube. The period right after you finish your chair yoga practice is ideal for meditation. You did an excellent job of creating the ideal environment for your workout. It is not difficult at all to make the change.

# Volunteering

Participating in volunteer work is the most selfless action one can do. That is really how it should be interpreted. What exactly am I trying to convey by saying that? I will explain it more. When we decide to volunteer for anything, we almost always have someone or something in mind that we want to assist, whether it be a person, a cause, a movement, or an organization. If we were to make such an assumption, we would be entirely correct. To assist another person without being required to do so or in exchange for payment is almost always received with gratitude. In addition, there are crucial advantages to the volunteer's mental and physical health that come along with volunteering, mainly when the volunteer is an older person. According to research by the National Institute on Aging, engaging in meaningful social activities such as volunteering may extend a person's life span, enhance mental health, and lower the chance of developing dementia. To quote yet another research, this one was carried out by the Corporation for National and Community Service. It was found that persons over the age of sixty who participated in volunteer work reported greater levels of general well-being than those who did not participate in volunteer work. Simply said, we get an incredible amount more from the act of volunteering than the people or organizations who ultimately benefit from our work.

Discovering a cause vital to oneself is, in my opinion, the most critical factor in having a satisfying experience when volunteering. One way to lead a purpose-driven life is to look for opportunities to teach or share the skills, knowledge, or interests you have developed through time with others. As I ponder this topic, a few specific instances of individuals who have benefited from their participation in volunteer work immediately come to me.

Mandy is well into her late sixties and has been retired for some time. However, she deeply appreciates the French language and culture, having majored in French in college. She visits a community center weekly to teach a class of older citizens the French language. Sharing her enthusiasm brings her a lot of joy, and she beams with pride whenever one of the members of her group achieves a milestone.

Gorge, now retired from the legal profession, donates his time at the Legal Aid Society in New York City once per week. When he can help a person in need, he feels like the happiest person in the world.

SCORE is an organization that benefits from Bred's expertise as a former company entrepreneur who gives his time there. It is the most extensive network of volunteer, professional business mentors in the country, and its primary mission is to assist individuals in launching their own companies. Fred has a lot of success in his life and is happy to be able to help others.

My uncle Bill went away when he was ninety-six years old and is the subject of my most heartfelt volunteer memory. Up until two weeks, before he passed away, he volunteered at the Veterans Affairs hospital in Seminole, Florida, for a total of two days per week. This was something that he had been doing for the last twenty years. Bill was a soldier of World War II, and the event had a significant and lasting impact on him. He was compelled to act because he felt compelled to assist soldiers who had been wounded in other conflicts that followed the "big one." Nothing could stop Bill from fulfilling his pledge of working two days weekly. He fought cancer multiple times and maintained his appointments at the VA hospital throughout his treatment. He was a model for me to follow in terms of giving back, passing on favors, and experiencing the transformative power of humanity.

# Connection to both the community and society

Social support and social integration are two crucial characteristics of our social environments that contribute to our overall health, according to a study by Sheldon Cohen of Carnegie Mellon University. In this section, I will concentrate on the component of community connectedness known as integration. How we go about our daily lives undergoes profound changes when we approach our senior years. Our children are now adults and have long since left the house. Because we may be retiring, we will no longer interact with our former coworkers regularly. Our habits, some of which we have followed for decades, are no longer practiced by us. Some people are excited about their newly discovered "freedom" from their jobs and families. Still, a far more significant number of people are essentially in mourning for a previous life that was rich with meaning and obligations. If we do not find a new way to live our lives in a manner that brings us joy, we are at risk for clinical depression, increased body fat, and worsening health. Most of you reading this book have successfully made the change, and you have robust support from your friends, family, and community. I do not doubt that you can provide me with some good instances of the therapeutic potential of the community. I want to provide some assistance to those of you who have had trouble locating a community activity that is a good fit for you and the things you are interested in doing.

Participating in a workout class offers physical benefits and essential connections to the community. Seniors are perfect candidates for the Silver Sneakers program. It is a benefit often included with Medicare or Medicare supplemental insurance and is accessible in every nation and region. The same group of individuals attends the courses frequently and form relationships before, during, and after the program. For example, my mother, who is ninety-four years old and lives in Largo, Florida, goes to a Silver Sneakers session three times a week. Her other students assist her in setting up her chair and dumbbells in the classroom. The instructor celebrated her ninety-fourth birthday by bringing a cake to school for her students to enjoy on that particular day. That is what we call community!

There are several entry points available to join various organizations. For example, I am a part of a knitting circle and a reading club. Reading and knitting are two of my favorite hobbies, but getting together with my two groups of friends provides me with much more happiness than finishing a book or a sweater. I adore and am nourished by the interactions with other people.

Think about those who play golf. It is possible to form deep social ties. Likewise, players that participate in card games like Bridge and Poker often get together to bond through their mutual enthusiasm for the activity.

What if you aren't the kind to "join in" on things? Now that we've established that, maybe it's time to give it a go. Attend a course at the community college in your area. Acquire some new linguistic skills. Master the skill of playing an instrument. Do you play pool? Bowl? Join a league. Come up with something! You should look for more than one item. It will improve your overall well-being and make you feel more robust and supported.

# Calming Down

## The Palming

This method requires that you take a seat.

Put down the spectacles and look around.

You may rub your hands together until you feel the warmth.

Put your hands together in a cupped position and put them over your eyes so that you can feel the warmth of your hands on your eyes.

Your eyes may be open or closed, whatever seems most comfortable to you at the moment.

Hold for anywhere between one and five minutes.

Warning: It is essential to avoid exerting any

pressure on your eyeballs at any point throughout this process.

Benefits: Feels friendly and calming.

# Rest and Repose at the End

The method calls for you to loosen up your hands by placing them on your lap.

Relax your entire body and enjoy the moment.

You should close your eyes and concentrate on breathing calmly and collectedly.

After you have completed this step, you should now gently open your eyes and move your fingers and toes.

If you want to prevent feeling dizzy when you get up from your chair, be sure you do it slowly and deliberately.

I hope you have an excellent remainder of your day.

Hold for up to five minutes for maximum effect.

There is no need to take any precautions since everyone may benefit from relaxing.

Benefits:

➤ Feels nice.

➤ Calming.

➤ Provides your body with the opportunity to begin assimilating the benefits of your yoga practice.

I have high hopes that you have found this sequence helpful as a practice in and of itself and as a starting point to enthuse you to develop your chair routines. Adding activity to your life or sharing it with others is a great gift, and I'm thankful for the opportunity to impart this knowledge to others since it gives me the chance to do any of those things.

If you liked what you read, feel free to leave a review                    on                    Amazon.

# Other books by Judith

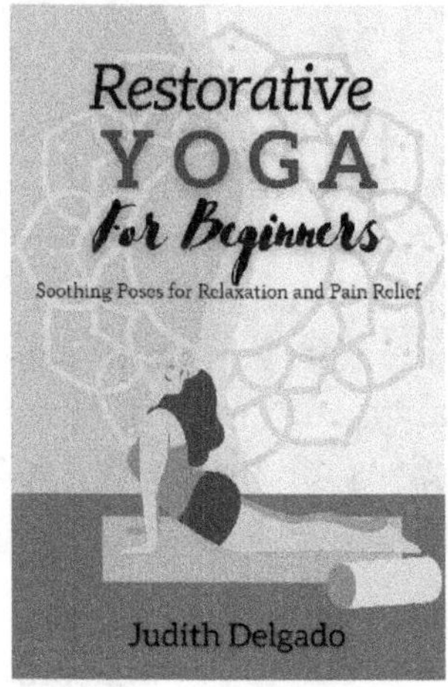

*Restorative Yoga for Beginners: Soothing Poses for Relaxation and Pain Relief*

It takes less than an hour a day to start relieving your mind and body from anxiety, past traumas, and unnecessary pain. Are you ready to deeply heal and start sensing your body like never before?

*If that is your case, this is the beginner's path you were looking for.*

With simple poses in supported positions, restorative yoga encourages deep relaxation so your body—as well as your mind—can enter a state of pure peace, even if this is your very first time approaching yoga.